AF367116

Clinical Trial Manager

-

The Comprehensive Guide

by

VIRUTI SHIVAN

Masters in Clinical Psychology (Major)

"In books, as in life, it's not the size or looks but the content that matters."

DISCLAIMER: The information in this book is provided for general informational purposes only and is not intended as professional advice. Although every effort has been made to ensure the accuracy and completeness of the information, the author and publisher do not assume responsibility for errors, inaccuracies, omissions, inconsistencies, or the impact of future advancements or updates in technology and information. This book is not a substitute for proper training, diagnosis, treatment, or guidance from qualified professionals. Readers are encouraged to consult experts in the relevant fields and independently verify the information when necessary. Any slights of people, places, or organizations are unintentional and purely coincidental.

Introduction

Welcome to "Clinical Trial Manager - The Comprehensive Guide," a pivotal resource designed to navigate the multifaceted world of clinical research management. This guide stands as a testament to the critical role that clinical trial managers play in the advancement of medical science and patient care. The journey of a clinical trial from conception to conclusion is intricate and fraught with challenges, yet it is undeniably rewarding. Through this book, we aim to equip you with the knowledge, skills, and insights necessary to lead successful clinical trials, thereby contributing significantly to medical research and innovation.

The Role of the Clinical Trial Manager

At the heart of every clinical trial is the Clinical Trial Manager (CTM), whose leadership and vision drive the project forward. The CTM is responsible for overseeing the planning, execution, and management of the trial, ensuring adherence to regulatory requirements, and maintaining ethical standards. This role requires a unique blend of scientific understanding, project management acumen, and interpersonal skills to navigate the complexities of clinical research effectively.

Navigating the Guide

This guide is structured to provide a comprehensive overview of clinical trial management, starting with the foundational aspects of clinical trials, including regulatory frameworks and ethical considerations. Each chapter is meticulously crafted to delve into the various facets of clinical trial management, from designing a trial and managing budgets to ensuring regulatory compliance and leveraging technology. The chapters include practical exercises to reinforce learning and application of the concepts discussed.

The journey through this guide is akin to the journey of managing a clinical trial. It begins with laying the groundwork and understanding the framework within which clinical trials operate. As we progress, we delve deeper into the strategic and operational aspects of trial management, addressing the challenges and opportunities that clinical trial managers face.

Emphasis on Ethics and Compliance

Ethical considerations and regulatory compliance form the backbone of clinical trial management. This guide emphasizes the importance of upholding ethical standards and adhering to regulatory requirements to ensure the integrity of the trial and the safety of participants. Through real-world examples and hypothetical scenarios, we explore the ethical dilemmas and regulatory challenges that may arise and provide strategies for navigating these complexities.

The Future of Clinical Trial Management

The landscape of clinical research is ever-evolving, with technological advancements and regulatory changes shaping the future of clinical trials. This guide also looks ahead, discussing the innovations in trial design and management that are likely to impact the field. We envision a future where clinical trial managers are not only adept at managing the trials of today but are also prepared to embrace the trials of tomorrow.

As you embark on this journey through "Clinical Trial Manager - The Comprehensive Guide," we invite you to engage with the material actively, reflect on the scenarios presented, and envision yourself applying these principles and strategies in real-world clinical trials. This guide is more than just a book; it is a companion on your path to becoming an effective and innovative clinical trial manager.

Chapter 1: The Foundation of Clinical Trial Management

1.1 Overview of Clinical Trials

Clinical trials are the cornerstone of medical research, providing essential data on the safety and efficacy of new treatments, interventions, and diagnostics. These rigorously controlled studies are the final step in a long process of research and development, designed to ensure that medical advancements are both safe for patients and effective in treating, preventing, or diagnosing diseases.

At their core, clinical trials are structured around phases, each with a specific purpose and set of objectives. Phase I trials focus on assessing the safety of a new intervention in a small group of participants. Phase II expands the focus to evaluate efficacy and further assess safety in a larger group. Phase III trials compare the new intervention against the current standard of care in a much larger population, providing the robust data needed for regulatory approval. Finally, Phase IV trials, conducted after approval, monitor the intervention's long-term effectiveness and impact in the general population.

The design of a clinical trial is critical to its success. It involves determining the study's objectives, endpoints, and methodology, including how participants are selected and allocated to different study groups. Randomized controlled trials (RCTs), considered the gold standard, randomly assign participants to the intervention or control group to minimize bias and provide the most reliable evidence of an intervention's effect.

Ethical considerations are paramount in clinical trials, governed by principles such as respect for persons, beneficence, and justice. These principles ensure that participants are treated with dignity, that the benefits of research outweigh the risks, and that the burdens and benefits of research are distributed fairly. Informed consent is a critical process, ensuring that participants understand the trial's nature, their role in it, and the potential risks and benefits before agreeing to take part.

Regulatory frameworks play a vital role in the oversight of clinical trials, ensuring that they are conducted in accordance with ethical principles and scientific standards. In the United States, the Food and Drug Administration (FDA) oversees clinical trials, while in Europe, the European Medicines Agency (EMA) fulfills a similar role. These agencies evaluate the scientific validity of trial protocols, monitor safety data, and ultimately decide whether a new intervention should be approved for public use.

The management of a clinical trial is a complex endeavor, requiring coordination among diverse stakeholders, including researchers, participants, regulatory authorities, and sponsors. Clinical Trial Managers (CTMs) are at the helm of this process, responsible for ensuring that trials are conducted efficiently, ethically, and in compliance with all regulatory requirements.

They oversee the planning, execution, and closeout of the trial, managing everything from budgeting and personnel to data collection and analysis.

In summary, clinical trials are a vital part of the medical research process, providing the data necessary to bring new treatments from the laboratory to the clinic. The successful management of these trials requires a deep understanding of their design, ethical considerations, and regulatory requirements—a foundation that is essential for anyone involved in the field of clinical trial management.

1.2 Key Regulatory Frameworks and Ethical Considerations

In the realm of clinical trials, adherence to rigorous regulatory frameworks and ethical considerations is paramount. These guidelines and principles ensure the safety, rights, and well-being of participants while maintaining the integrity and credibility of the research. The landscape of these frameworks is vast, shaped by historical milestones that have underscored the importance of ethical conduct in medical research.

At the heart of the regulatory environment are sets of rules and standards that govern the conduct of clinical trials globally. These frameworks outline the processes for trial approval, conduct, monitoring, reporting, and publication of results. They aim to ensure that all clinical research meets the highest standards of safety, efficacy, and ethical responsibility. The guidelines specify requirements for trial design, participant consent, data management, and the responsibilities of trial sponsors and investigators.

Ethical considerations in clinical trials are grounded in universally recognized principles. The first principle emphasizes respect for individuals, acknowledging their autonomy and the need to protect those with diminished autonomy. This principle underscores the importance of informed consent, ensuring that participants are fully aware of the trial's nature, its potential risks and benefits, and their rights as participants, including the right to withdraw at any time without penalty.

The second principle, beneficence, compels researchers to maximize benefits and minimize harms. This involves conducting a thorough risk-benefit analysis to ensure that the potential benefits of the research justify any risks involved. The aim is to protect participants from harm and ensure their welfare is a primary consideration throughout the trial process.

Justice, the third principle, relates to the equitable selection and treatment of participants. It addresses issues of fairness in bearing the burdens and enjoying the benefits of research, ensuring that no group is unfairly burdened or excluded from the potential benefits of the research.

In addition to these ethical pillars, the concept of voluntary participation is crucial. It emphasizes that participation in clinical trials should be a voluntary act, free from coercion or undue influence. Participants must have the freedom to choose whether to participate or continue in a trial based on a clear understanding of their involvement.

These regulatory frameworks and ethical principles are not static; they evolve in response to emerging challenges, advancements in science and medicine, and societal values. The ongoing dialogue between regulatory bodies, researchers, participants, and society is vital in shaping an ethical and effective research environment that respects the dignity and rights of individuals while advancing medical knowledge.

In essence, the ethical and regulatory landscape of clinical trials serves as a foundation for conducting research that is not only scientifically sound but also morally responsible. This dual commitment ensures that clinical trials can continue to play a critical role in advancing medical science and improving patient care, upholding the highest standards of integrity and respect for human dignity.

1.3 Roles and Responsibilities of a Clinical Trial Manager

The role of a Clinical Trial Manager (CTM) is pivotal in the orchestration of clinical trials, embodying a multifaceted set of responsibilities that ensure the smooth execution and integrity of the trial from inception to conclusion. This position demands a unique blend of scientific knowledge, project management skills, and ethical vigilance, serving as the linchpin that holds the complex web of clinical trial activities together.

Leadership and Team Management

A CTM is primarily responsible for leading the clinical trial team, fostering a collaborative environment where communication is clear, and objectives are understood by all team members. This leadership role involves coordinating tasks among diverse team members, including biostatisticians, clinical researchers, data managers, and health care professionals, ensuring that each individual's work aligns with the trial's objectives and timelines.

Project Planning and Execution

Effective project management is at the core of a CTM's responsibilities. This involves meticulous planning, including defining the scope of the trial, setting realistic timelines, and allocating resources efficiently. The CTM must ensure that the trial is executed according to the protocol, within budget, and in compliance with regulatory requirements, adjusting strategies as needed to address challenges that arise during the trial.

Regulatory Compliance and Documentation

Ensuring compliance with regulatory frameworks is a critical responsibility. The CTM navigates complex regulatory landscapes, ensuring that all aspects of the trial adhere to relevant guidelines and laws. This includes preparing and submitting regulatory documents, obtaining necessary approvals, and ensuring that the trial's conduct is ethically sound. Maintaining accurate and comprehensive documentation is essential for audit readiness and for providing clear evidence of compliance and the integrity of the trial data.

Participant Safety and Communication

The safety of trial participants is paramount. The CTM oversees the monitoring of participant safety, ensuring that adverse events are reported promptly and that necessary actions are taken to mitigate risks. Effective communication with participants is also crucial, ensuring they are fully informed about the trial, their rights, and what participation involves.

Data Management and Quality Assurance

Overseeing data management processes to ensure the accuracy, completeness, and confidentiality of trial data is another key responsibility. This includes implementing systems for data collection, storage, and analysis that uphold the highest standards of data integrity. The CTM also plays a crucial role in quality assurance, developing and enforcing quality control measures to ensure that all aspects of the trial meet predefined standards of excellence.

Stakeholder Engagement

Engaging with stakeholders, including sponsors, regulatory bodies, and patient advocacy groups, is a continuous responsibility. The CTM acts as the primary liaison, communicating trial progress, addressing concerns, and ensuring that stakeholder expectations are managed effectively.

In conclusion, the role of a Clinical Trial Manager is both challenging and rewarding, requiring a dynamic set of skills to manage the complexities of clinical trials. Through effective leadership, meticulous planning, and unwavering commitment to ethical standards, the CTM ensures that clinical trials are conducted efficiently, safely, and with the highest level of integrity, ultimately contributing to the advancement of medical science and patient care.

1.4 Exercise: 10 MCQs with Answers at the End

Multiple Choice Questions:

1. What is the primary purpose of Phase I clinical trials?

   - A) To assess the long-term side effects of a treatment.

   - B) To determine the efficacy of a treatment.

- C) To assess the safety and dosage of a treatment.

- D) To compare the new treatment with current standards.

2. Which principle emphasizes the need for researchers to maximize benefits and minimize harms in clinical trials?

   - A) Respect for persons

   - B) Beneficence

   - C) Justice

   - D) Informed consent

3. What is the role of an Institutional Review Board (IRB) in clinical trials?

   - A) To fund the clinical trial

   - B) To market the pharmaceutical products

   - C) To oversee the ethical aspects of the study

   - D) To recruit participants for the study

4. Which phase of clinical trials is primarily focused on evaluating the efficacy of an intervention?

   - A) Phase I

   - B) Phase II

   - C) Phase III

   - D) Phase IV

5. Informed consent in clinical trials ensures that:

   - A) Participants are compensated for their time.

   - B) Participants are aware of the trial details and voluntarily agree to partake.

   - C) All participants receive the treatment being tested.

   - D) The trial will definitely lead to new treatments being available.

6. Which of the following best describes the responsibilities of a Clinical Trial Manager?

   - A) Patient recruitment only

   - B) Data analysis only

   - C) Overseeing trial execution, ensuring regulatory compliance, and managing the trial team

   - D) Providing medical care to trial participants

7. A randomized controlled trial is considered the gold standard because it:

   - A) Takes the least time to complete.

   - B) Costs less than other types of trials.

   - C) Minimizes bias and provides the most reliable evidence of an intervention's effect.

   - D) Does not require informed consent.

8. Ethical considerations in clinical trials are based on all the following principles EXCEPT:

   - A) Autonomy

   - B) Maleficence

   - C) Beneficence

   - D) Justice

9. The main goal of Phase IV clinical trials is to:

   - A) Determine the treatment's dosage.

   - B) Assess the treatment's safety in a small group of volunteers.

   - C) Evaluate the treatment's efficacy in a larger group of patients.

   - D) Monitor the treatment's long-term effectiveness and impact.

10. Regulatory frameworks in clinical trials aim to:

   - A) Ensure the trial is conducted without the need for documentation.

   - B) Eliminate the necessity for participant consent.

   - C) Guarantee that the trial adheres to ethical principles and scientific standards.

   - D) Allow trials to proceed without monitoring or audits.

Answers:

1. C) To assess the safety and dosage of a treatment.

2. B) Beneficence

3. C) To oversee the ethical aspects of the study

4. B) Phase II

5. B) Participants are aware of the trial details and voluntarily agree to partake.

6. C) Overseeing trial execution, ensuring regulatory compliance, and managing the trial team

7. C) Minimizes bias and provides the most reliable evidence of an intervention's effect.

8. B) Maleficence

9. D) Monitor the treatment's long-term effectiveness and impact.

10. C) Guarantee that the trial adheres to ethical principles and scientific standards.

Chapter 2: Designing a Clinical Trial

2.1 Defining Objectives and Endpoints

The foundation of a successful clinical trial lies in its design, starting with a clear definition of its objectives and endpoints. This initial step is crucial as it guides every subsequent decision in the trial process, from selecting the right participants to choosing the most effective data analysis techniques.

Objectives:

The objectives of a clinical trial articulate the questions the trial seeks to answer. They are the overarching goals that guide the direction of the research. Objectives can be broad, such as determining the efficacy of a new intervention compared to a standard treatment, or they can be specific, like assessing the impact of a treatment on a particular symptom or biomarker. Well-defined objectives are SMART: Specific, Measurable, Achievable, Relevant, and Time-bound. This precision ensures that the trial is designed efficiently and can achieve its goals within the constraints of time, budget, and resources.

Endpoints:

Endpoints are specific outcomes used to measure whether the objectives of the trial have been met. They provide a clear metric for evaluating the effectiveness and safety of the intervention being studied. Endpoints can be classified into primary and secondary types, with primary endpoints directly related to the main objective of the trial. For example, in a trial testing a new medication for hypertension, a primary endpoint could be the reduction in systolic blood pressure among participants. Secondary endpoints, while also important, might include the medication's effects on cholesterol levels or quality of life measures.

Choosing the right endpoints is critical. They must be clinically meaningful, measurable, and susceptible to change as a result of the intervention. The selection of endpoints often involves a delicate balance between scientific rigor and practical considerations, such as the availability of reliable measurement methods and the time frame within which changes can realistically be observed.

Clinical and Surrogate Endpoints:

Endpoints can be further categorized into clinical endpoints and surrogate endpoints. Clinical endpoints are direct measures of how a patient feels, functions, or survives. These are the most straightforward and convincing indicators of the intervention's impact but can require large sample sizes and long follow-up periods. Surrogate endpoints, on the other hand, are indirect measures expected to predict clinical benefits, such as biomarkers or physical signs. They can expedite trials and reduce costs but carry the risk of not accurately predicting clinical outcomes.

Composite Endpoints:

In some trials, especially those addressing complex diseases, composite endpoints that combine several individual outcomes into a single measure are used. These can increase the trial's efficiency by capturing multiple aspects of the intervention's effect. However, they must be chosen and interpreted with care to avoid diluting important findings or obscuring adverse effects.

In conclusion, defining objectives and endpoints with precision and care is the first and perhaps most crucial step in designing a clinical trial. This process sets the stage for the trial's success, ensuring that the research is focused, meaningful, and capable of advancing medical knowledge and patient care.

2.2 Selecting Appropriate Study Designs

The selection of an appropriate study design is a pivotal decision in the development of a clinical trial, determining the trial's structure, the type of data collected, and the methods of analysis. This decision shapes how effectively the trial can answer its research questions and meet its objectives. Various designs offer different strengths and limitations, and choosing the right one depends on the specific goals of the trial, the nature of the intervention, and the practical considerations of conducting the study.

Randomized Controlled Trials (RCTs):

RCTs are the gold standard of clinical trial designs, minimizing bias by randomly assigning participants to either the intervention group or the control group. This randomization ensures that any differences observed between the groups can be attributed to the intervention itself rather than pre-existing differences among participants. RCTs can be blinded or double-blinded to further reduce bias by preventing participants, and sometimes researchers, from knowing which group they are in, thus ensuring that the outcomes are not influenced by expectations.

Cohort Studies:

Cohort studies follow a group of people over time to observe outcomes under different exposures. While not typically used for interventional trials, they are valuable in observational research, especially for assessing long-term or rare outcomes. Cohort studies can be prospective, starting in the present and following participants into the future, or retrospective, using existing records to follow participants' histories backward in time.

Case-Control Studies:

Case-control studies are retrospective, observational studies that start with an outcome (such as a disease) and work backward to ascertain exposures. They compare individuals with the condition (cases) to those without (controls) to identify factors that may contribute to the outcome. This design is particularly useful for studying rare conditions or diseases with long latency periods but is less reliable for determining causality.

Cross-Sectional Studies:

Cross-sectional studies examine a population at a single point in time, providing a "snapshot" of the frequency and characteristics of a disease, condition, or other health-related variables. While quick and relatively inexpensive, these studies cannot establish causality or the sequence of events, limiting their use in interventional research.

Adaptive Designs:

Adaptive designs allow modifications to the trial's procedures or hypotheses based on interim data without compromising the integrity of the study. These designs can include adjustments to sample size, dosing schedules, or even the addition or removal of treatment arms. Adaptive designs offer flexibility and efficiency, especially in early-phase trials, but require careful planning and transparent protocols to ensure validity and prevent bias.

Factorial Designs:

Factorial designs test the effect of multiple interventions simultaneously by assigning participants to all possible combinations of the interventions being studied. This design can efficiently assess interactions between treatments and is particularly useful when investigating the combined effect of two or more interventions.

Cluster Randomized Trials:

In cluster randomized trials, groups or clusters of participants, rather than individual participants, are randomly assigned to intervention or control conditions. This design is useful when the intervention is delivered at the group level or when individual randomization is impractical or impossible.

Selecting the right study design is a critical step that influences the validity, reliability, and generalizability of the trial's findings. The choice of design should be driven by the research question, the ethical considerations, and the logistical aspects of conducting the study, ensuring that the chosen design can robustly and efficiently achieve the trial's objectives.

2.3 Considerations for Trial Protocols

A clinical trial protocol is a detailed plan that outlines the rationale, objectives, design, methodology, statistical considerations, and organization of a trial. It serves as a guide for conducting the study and ensures that the research is performed consistently across different locations and by various investigators. Developing a robust protocol is crucial for the success of a clinical trial, as it addresses several key considerations that impact the trial's validity, reliability, and ethical compliance.

Rationale and Objectives:

The protocol must begin with a clear statement of the research question, providing the scientific background and rationale for the trial. This section explains why the study is necessary, citing previous research and identifying gaps in knowledge that the current trial aims to address. Objectives should be specific, measurable, achievable, relevant, and time-bound (SMART), clearly stating what the trial intends to accomplish.

Trial Design:

The choice of trial design is critical and should be justified in the protocol. This includes deciding on the type of trial (e.g., randomized controlled trial, cohort study, case-control study), the nature of the control group, blinding mechanisms, and any stratification or clustering. The design section should also outline the criteria for participant inclusion and exclusion, ensuring that the study population is appropriately defined and that the trial's findings will be generalizable to a broader population.

Interventions:

Detailed descriptions of the interventions to be tested, including the dose, frequency, duration, and route of administration, are essential. For trials testing more than one intervention or comparing interventions to a control, the rationale for each choice must be clearly explained. The protocol should also specify any concomitant treatments allowed or prohibited during the trial.

Outcomes:

Primary and secondary outcomes should be clearly defined, including how and when they will be measured. The choice of outcomes should reflect the trial's objectives and be clinically meaningful. The protocol must detail the methods used to assess each outcome, including any tools or instruments employed and their validity and reliability.

Participant Recruitment and Consent:

The protocol should outline the strategies for participant recruitment, ensuring that the process is fair and equitable. It must also describe the informed consent process, emphasizing how participants will be informed about the trial's purpose, potential risks and benefits, and their rights, including the right to withdraw from the study at any time.

Data Management and Statistical Analysis:

This section details how data will be collected, stored, and analyzed, ensuring the confidentiality and integrity of participant information. It should include the statistical methods to be used for analyzing the trial's outcomes, criteria for data inclusion or exclusion, and plans for handling missing data. The protocol should also specify any interim analyses or stopping rules for the trial.

Ethical Considerations:

The protocol must address ethical issues related to the trial, including how the study adheres to ethical guidelines and any potential conflicts of interest. It should describe the process for obtaining ethical approval from institutional review boards or ethics committees and outline the measures taken to minimize risks and protect participant welfare.

Monitoring and Quality Assurance:

Plans for monitoring the trial's conduct and ensuring quality control and assurance should be included. This includes the roles and responsibilities of the monitoring committee, data safety monitoring board, and any external auditors. The protocol should also describe the procedures for reporting adverse events and how protocol deviations will be managed.

A well-constructed protocol is fundamental to the success of a clinical trial, guiding every aspect of its implementation and ensuring that the study is conducted with rigor, ethical integrity, and respect for participant rights. It forms the basis for regulatory approval, participant recruitment, and the ultimate credibility and utility of the trial's findings.

2.4 Exercise: 10 MCQs with Answers at the End

Multiple Choice Questions:

1. What is the primary purpose of a clinical trial protocol?

   - A) To market the intervention to potential investors

   - B) To detail the study plan, including design, objectives, and methodology

- C) To recruit participants for the study

- D) To predict the outcomes of the trial

2. Which aspect of a trial protocol defines the study population?

- A) Data management plan

- B) Inclusion and exclusion criteria

- C) Statistical analysis plan

- D) Ethical considerations

3. What is the significance of randomization in clinical trial design?

- A) It ensures that the trial results are profitable.

- B) It minimizes bias by distributing known and unknown factors evenly between groups.

- C) It eliminates the need for a control group.

- D) It guarantees that the intervention will be successful.

4. Which of the following best describes blinding in clinical trials?

- A) Ensuring that all trials are conducted in secret

- B) Preventing participants from leaving the trial early

- C) Keeping participants, and sometimes researchers, unaware of group assignments

- D) Making all trial data publicly available immediately

5. What is the purpose of defining primary and secondary outcomes in a trial protocol?

   - A) To confuse competitors

   - B) To determine the dosage of the intervention

   - C) To specify what the trial aims to measure and analyze

   - D) To increase the trial's duration unnecessarily

6. Why is the informed consent process crucial in clinical trials?

   - A) It guarantees a high participant retention rate.

   - B) It ensures participants are fully aware of the trial details and agree to partake voluntarily.

   - C) It allows researchers to modify the protocol without approval.

   - D) It helps in speeding up the recruitment process.

7. In a trial protocol, the statistical analysis plan is important because:

   - A) It outlines how to promote the trial on social media.

   - B) It specifies how data will be analyzed to assess the trial's outcomes.

   - C) It determines the financial compensation for participants.

   - D) It lists the potential sponsors of the trial.

8. Ethical considerations in a trial protocol are primarily concerned with:

  - A) Ensuring the trial is profitable.

  - B) Maximizing the publication potential of the trial results.

 - C) Protecting participant welfare and ensuring ethical conduct.

  - D) Selecting trial locations based on convenience.

9. The inclusion and exclusion criteria in a trial protocol are designed to:

  - A) Ensure the trial results favor the intervention.

  - B) Define the specific population for which the trial's findings will be applicable.

  - C) Exclude individuals who do not consent to participate.

  - D) Simplify data analysis by reducing variability.

10. What role does the data management plan play in a clinical trial protocol?

  - A) It specifies the color scheme for the trial's promotional materials.

  - B) It ensures the confidentiality and integrity of trial data.

  - C) It details the trial's social media strategy.

  - D) It outlines the daily schedule for trial participants.

Answers:

1. B) To detail the study plan, including design, objectives, and methodology

2. B) Inclusion and exclusion criteria

3. B) It minimizes bias by distributing known and unknown factors evenly between groups.

4. C) Keeping participants, and sometimes researchers, unaware of group assignments

5. C) To specify what the trial aims to measure and analyze

6. B) It ensures participants are fully aware of the trial details and agree to partake voluntarily.

7. B) It specifies how data will be analyzed to assess the trial's outcomes.

8. C) Protecting participant welfare and ensuring ethical conduct.

9. B) Define the specific population for which the trial's findings will be applicable.

10. B) It ensures the confidentiality and integrity of trial data.

Chapter 3: Budgeting and Funding

3.1 Principles of Budgeting for Clinical Trials

Budgeting for clinical trials is a complex and critical process that ensures the necessary resources are allocated efficiently to conduct the trial successfully. It involves estimating the financial resources required for all aspects of the trial, from inception to completion, while anticipating and mitigating potential financial risks. Here are the fundamental principles of budgeting for clinical trials:

Accurate Cost Estimation:

The cornerstone of effective budgeting is the accurate estimation of costs. This includes direct costs such as participant recruitment, medical procedures, personnel, and equipment, as well as indirect costs like administrative support and facility overheads. It's crucial to perform a thorough cost analysis, considering the trial's scope, duration, and specific needs to prevent budget overruns.

Flexibility and Contingency Planning:

Clinical trials often face unforeseen challenges that can impact the budget, such as delays in recruitment, changes in regulatory requirements, or unexpected adverse events. Incorporating flexibility into the budget and having a contingency fund (typically 10-20% of the total budget) can help manage these uncertainties without compromising the trial's objectives.

Prioritization and Resource Allocation:

Given the limitations of funding, it's essential to prioritize spending based on the trial's critical needs and objectives. This means allocating resources efficiently, ensuring that key aspects of the trial, such as patient safety and data integrity, receive the necessary funding, while identifying areas where costs can be minimized without impacting the trial's success.

Transparent and Detailed Documentation:

Maintaining transparent and detailed documentation of all budgeting decisions and expenditures is crucial for financial accountability and reporting. This documentation facilitates effective communication with sponsors, regulatory bodies, and other stakeholders, and can be invaluable in case of audits or financial reviews.

Ongoing Monitoring and Review:

The budget should be monitored continuously throughout the trial, with regular reviews to compare actual spending against the budget. This allows for timely adjustments in response to deviations, ensuring that the trial remains financially viable without sacrificing quality or compliance.

Understanding Funding Sources:

Identifying and securing funding is a critical component of the budgeting process. Sources of funding can vary widely, including governmental grants, industry sponsors, nonprofit organizations, and institutional funds. Understanding the requirements and constraints of each funding source, such as restrictions on spending or reporting obligations, is essential for successful budget management.

Cost Recovery and Sustainability:

For trials funded by industry sponsors or where there is potential for commercialization, developing a cost recovery plan is essential. This involves negotiating contracts that ensure the trial's costs are covered and considering long-term sustainability, such as the potential for funding future phases of the research.

Stakeholder Engagement:

Engaging with all stakeholders, including sponsors, institutional finance departments, and clinical teams, in the budgeting process ensures that all costs are considered and that the budget aligns with the trial's objectives and stakeholder expectations.

In conclusion, effective budgeting for clinical trials requires a comprehensive, flexible, and proactive approach to financial planning. By adhering to these principles, trial managers can ensure that the trial is conducted efficiently, with adequate resources to achieve its objectives, while navigating the financial uncertainties inherent in clinical research.

3.2 Identifying and Securing Funding Sources

Identifying and securing funding is a crucial step in the execution of clinical trials, necessitating a strategic approach to explore and tap into various potential sources. The landscape of funding is diverse, offering multiple avenues through which clinical trials can receive the financial backing needed to commence and successfully reach completion. Here's a comprehensive guide to navigating this critical phase:

Government Grants and Public Funding:

Numerous government agencies globally allocate funds specifically for medical research, including clinical trials. These grants are highly competitive and require detailed proposals that highlight the study's significance, potential impact, and scientific merit. Applying for government grants often involves a rigorous review process but provides substantial funding without the expectation of profit return, allowing for more independent research.

Pharmaceutical and Biotechnology Companies:

Industry sponsorship is a significant source of funding for clinical trials, particularly those testing new drugs, devices, or therapies. Collaborating with these companies often means access to substantial resources and cutting-edge technologies. However, it's crucial to establish clear agreements regarding the study's design, data ownership, publication rights, and potential conflicts of interest to maintain scientific integrity and independence.

Non-Profit Organizations and Foundations:

Many non-profit organizations, including disease-specific foundations, are dedicated to advancing research in particular areas of health and medicine. These organizations might provide grants or funding for clinical trials that align with their mission. Funding from these sources can also enhance the trial's visibility and public engagement, aiding recruitment and community support.

Academic and Research Institutions:

Institutions often allocate funds for research initiatives, including clinical trials conducted by their staff. These funds can be an excellent way to cover pilot studies or smaller-scale research projects, which can then leverage results to secure larger grants. Institutional support may also include access to facilities, administrative assistance, and other in-kind contributions.

Crowdfunding and Philanthropy:

With the rise of digital platforms, crowdfunding has emerged as a viable option for securing funds for clinical trials. By appealing directly to the public, researchers can raise awareness and small contributions from a broad audience. Additionally, philanthropic donations from individuals or entities with an interest in advancing medical research can provide substantial funding, often with fewer restrictions than other sources.

Collaborative Partnerships and Consortia:

Joining forces with other research groups or forming consortia can open up opportunities for shared funding from sources interested in larger, multi-center studies. These partnerships can also facilitate resource sharing, reducing the overall cost burden for individual participants.

Strategies for Securing Funding:

- **Compelling Proposals:** Crafting well-written, compelling proposals that clearly articulate the trial's significance, design, and potential impact is crucial.

- **Networking:** Building relationships with potential funders and industry partners through conferences, seminars, and professional associations can increase visibility and open funding opportunities.

- **Transparency and Compliance:** Demonstrating a commitment to ethical research practices, participant safety, and data integrity can enhance credibility and attract funding.

- **Leveraging Preliminary Data:** Presenting strong preliminary data can make a compelling case for the feasibility and potential success of the trial, attracting more funding.

Identifying and securing funding for clinical trials requires a multifaceted approach, combining thorough research, strategic planning, and effective communication. By exploring a variety of funding sources and employing targeted strategies, researchers can secure the necessary financial support to advance medical science and improve patient care.

3.3 Financial Management and Oversight

Effective financial management and oversight are paramount in clinical trial operations, ensuring that resources are used efficiently and that the trial remains within budget while adhering to the highest standards of ethical and scientific integrity. This aspect of clinical trial management encompasses a range of activities, from budgeting and accounting to financial reporting and auditing. Here are the key principles and practices involved in robust financial management and oversight of clinical trials:

Establishing a Dedicated Financial Management Team:

A specialized team or individual should be designated to handle the financial aspects of the trial, including budget creation, allocation of funds, monitoring expenditures, and financial reporting. This team works closely with the clinical trial manager and other stakeholders to ensure that financial operations align with the trial's objectives and regulatory requirements.

Developing a Detailed Budget:

Creating a comprehensive budget that accurately reflects all potential expenses is the foundation of effective financial management. This includes direct costs (e.g., personnel, equipment, participant compensation) and indirect costs (e.g., administrative support, facility overhead). A detailed budget facilitates negotiations with sponsors and helps in securing adequate funding.

Implementing Financial Controls:

Financial controls are mechanisms put in place to prevent overspending and financial fraud. This includes setting expenditure limits, requiring multiple approvals for significant expenses, and segregating duties among team members to prevent conflicts of interest. Regular financial reviews and audits further strengthen these controls by identifying and correcting discrepancies in a timely manner.

Monitoring and Reconciling Expenditures:

Continuous monitoring of expenditures against the budget allows for early detection of deviations and the implementation of corrective measures. Regular reconciliation of accounts ensures that all transactions are accounted for and that financial records accurately reflect the trial's financial status.

Ensuring Compliance with Financial Regulations and Sponsor Requirements:

Clinical trials must adhere to a complex set of financial regulations and sponsor requirements, including those related to participant compensation, tax obligations, and reporting standards. Financial management practices must ensure compliance with these requirements to avoid legal and financial penalties.

Financial Reporting and Communication:

Transparent and regular financial reporting to stakeholders, including sponsors, institutional review boards, and regulatory agencies, is essential for maintaining trust and accountability. These reports should provide a clear and accurate picture of the trial's financial health, including expenditures, remaining funds, and any financial risks or issues.

Planning for Financial Risks and Uncertainties:

Identifying potential financial risks, such as unexpected increases in costs or delays in funding disbursements, and developing contingency plans are crucial components of financial oversight. This may involve establishing an emergency fund or identifying alternative funding sources to ensure the trial can proceed as planned despite financial setbacks.

Closing and Final Financial Audit:

At the trial's conclusion, a final financial report and audit should be conducted to ensure that all funds have been used appropriately and that any remaining funds are dealt with according to the sponsor's guidelines and regulatory requirements. This final step ensures financial closure and compliance, facilitating the transition to post-trial activities or subsequent phases of research.

Effective financial management and oversight in clinical trials not only ensure the efficient use of resources but also contribute to the trial's integrity and credibility. By adhering to these principles and practices, trial managers can navigate the financial complexities of clinical research, safeguarding the trial's success and the advancement of medical science.

3.4 Exercise: 10 MCQs with Answers at the End

Multiple Choice Questions:

1. Which of the following is a primary component of financial management in clinical trials?

   - A) Developing a marketing strategy

   - B) Creating a detailed budget

   - C) Designing the trial logo

   - D) Organizing team-building events

2. Effective financial oversight in clinical trials includes:

   - A) Ignoring minor budget deviations

   - B) Implementing financial controls

   - C) Limiting financial reporting to annual updates

   - D) Allowing unrestricted access to funds

3. A detailed budget for a clinical trial should NOT include which of the following?

   - A) Indirect costs such as administrative support

   - B) Only the highest estimated costs to ensure a surplus

   - C) Direct costs such as personnel and equipment

   - D) Estimated participant compensation

4. Financial controls in clinical trials are used to:

   - A) Increase spending flexibility

   - B) Prevent overspending and financial fraud

   - C) Complicate the financial management process

   - D) Reduce transparency in financial reporting

5. Monitoring and reconciling expenditures in clinical trials helps to:

   - A) Avoid financial reviews and audits

   - B) Identify and correct discrepancies

- C) Eliminate the need for a detailed budget

- D) Increase the trial's duration unnecessarily

6. Ensuring compliance with financial regulations and sponsor requirements is crucial to:

    - A) Make the trial more appealing to potential participants

    - B) Avoid legal and financial penalties

    - C) Simplify the financial management process

    - D) Guarantee the success of the trial

7. Regular financial reporting to stakeholders is important for:

    - A) Reducing the frequency of team meetings

    - B) Maintaining trust and accountability

    - C) Decreasing transparency in the trial's operations

    - D) Ignoring financial risks and uncertainties

8. Planning for financial risks and uncertainties involves:

    - A) Assuming that all budget estimates are accurate

    - B) Establishing an emergency fund

    - C) Avoiding the identification of alternative funding sources

    - D) Increasing dependency on a single source of funding

9. The purpose of the final financial audit at the trial's conclusion is to ensure:

   - A) There are no remaining funds

   - B) All funds have been used appropriately

   - C) Future trials do not require audits

   - D) Financial reporting is no longer necessary

10. Financial management and oversight in clinical trials contribute to:

   - A) The complexity of trial design

   - B) The trial's integrity and credibility

   - C) Limiting stakeholder engagement

   - D) Reducing the need for a financial management team

Answers:

1. B) Creating a detailed budget

2. B) Implementing financial controls

3. B) Only the highest estimated costs to ensure a surplus

4. B) Prevent overspending and financial fraud

5. B) Identify and correct discrepancies

6. B) Avoid legal and financial penalties

7. B) Maintaining trust and accountability

8. B) Establishing an emergency fund

9. B) All funds have been used appropriately

10. B) The trial's integrity and credibility

Chapter 4: Site Selection and Management

4.1 Criteria for Choosing Trial Sites

Choosing the right sites for a clinical trial is a pivotal decision that can significantly impact the study's success. The selection process involves a thorough evaluation of potential sites against a set of criteria designed to ensure that the trial can be conducted efficiently, ethically, and effectively. Here are the key criteria to consider when choosing trial sites:

Experience and Expertise:

A site's experience in conducting clinical trials, especially those similar in nature to the planned study, is a crucial factor. Experienced sites are more likely to understand the nuances of trial protocols, patient management, and regulatory compliance. The expertise of the site's principal investigator and staff in the therapeutic area of the trial also plays a significant role in ensuring high-quality data and adherence to the trial protocol.

Patient Population:

Access to a suitable patient population that meets the trial's inclusion and exclusion criteria is essential. Sites should have a sufficient number of potential participants to meet enrollment targets and consider factors such as disease prevalence in the area, demographic diversity, and the potential for patient retention throughout the trial duration.

Infrastructure and Facilities:

The availability of appropriate infrastructure and facilities to support the trial's requirements is another critical consideration. This includes necessary equipment, laboratory services, and technology for data collection and management. The site should also have adequate space to conduct the trial and ensure the comfort and privacy of participants.

Regulatory and Ethical Compliance:

Sites must have a track record of compliance with regulatory requirements and ethical standards. This includes adherence to Good Clinical Practice (GCP) guidelines, timely reporting of adverse events, and the ability to obtain necessary approvals from institutional review boards or ethics committees.

Operational Efficiency:

The operational capabilities of the site, including staff availability, workload capacity, and management practices, influence the site's ability to meet the trial's timelines and budget. Efficient sites can significantly reduce delays in study startup, patient enrollment, and data collection processes.

Patient Recruitment and Retention Strategies:

Sites with effective patient recruitment and retention strategies are more likely to meet enrollment targets and minimize dropout rates. This includes having established networks for patient outreach, experience in patient education and engagement, and strategies to address common barriers to participation.

Data Quality and Integrity:

The ability of the site to collect and report high-quality, accurate data is paramount. This involves having trained personnel, robust data management systems, and a commitment to maintaining the integrity of the trial data.

Communication and Collaboration:

Effective communication and collaboration between the trial sponsor, the site, and other stakeholders are essential for the smooth conduct of the trial. Sites that are responsive, transparent, and proactive in addressing issues are more likely to foster successful partnerships.

Geographical Location:

The geographical location of the site can affect patient access, investigator meetings, and the logistics of trial material shipments. Consideration should be given to sites that are easily accessible for participants and have reliable transportation and infrastructure.

In conclusion, selecting the right trial sites is a multifaceted process that requires careful consideration of various criteria. By prioritizing sites that demonstrate experience, patient access, operational efficiency, and a commitment to quality and ethical standards, sponsors can enhance the likelihood of trial success.

4.2 Site Initiation and Training

Site initiation and training are pivotal steps in the clinical trial process, laying the foundation for a trial's success by ensuring that each site is fully prepared to begin recruiting participants and conducting the study according to the protocol. This phase involves a series of coordinated activities aimed at equipping the site and its staff with the necessary information, tools, and procedures to carry out the trial effectively and ethically.

Site Initiation Visits:

The process typically begins with a site initiation visit (SIV), which is conducted by the clinical trial sponsor or a designated representative (often a clinical research associate). The primary objectives of the SIV are to:

- **Review the study protocol** with site staff to ensure a clear understanding of the study objectives, procedures, and responsibilities.

- **Verify site facilities and equipment** to ensure they meet the study requirements for conducting the trial and managing the data.

- **Confirm regulatory and ethical approvals** have been obtained and that the site is compliant with all local, national, and international regulations and guidelines governing clinical research.

- **Discuss recruitment strategies** to ensure the site has a plan for identifying, recruiting, and retaining participants in accordance with the study protocol.

Training for Site Staff:

Comprehensive training for all site staff involved in the trial is essential to maintain the quality and integrity of the study. Training topics include, but are not limited to:

- **Study-specific procedures and protocol**, focusing on critical elements such as consent processes, intervention administration, data collection, and adverse event reporting.

- **Good Clinical Practice (GCP)**, emphasizing the ethical and quality standards for designing, conducting, and reporting trials involving human subjects.

- **Data management systems**, including the use of electronic data capture systems, ensuring that staff are proficient in entering and managing study data accurately and securely.

- **Emergency procedures**, including how to handle adverse events, protocol deviations, and other unexpected situations.

Establishing Communication Channels:

Effective communication channels between the trial sponsor, site coordinators, and investigators are established during the site initiation phase. This includes setting up regular meetings, reporting schedules, and points of contact for trial-related inquiries, ensuring ongoing support and oversight throughout the trial.

Documenting and Finalizing Preparations:

All training activities, discussions, and site preparations are thoroughly documented during the site initiation visit. This documentation serves as a record of the site's readiness and commitment to follow the trial protocol and GCP standards. Once the site initiation process is complete, and all criteria are met, the site is officially authorized to start enrolling participants.

Site initiation and training are critical to a clinical trial's operational success, ensuring that sites are fully prepared, staff are well-trained, and the trial can be conducted consistently across locations. This meticulous preparation helps safeguard participant safety, data integrity, and overall study validity.

4.3 Monitoring Site Performance

Monitoring site performance is an essential component of clinical trial management, ensuring that each site adheres to the study protocol, complies with regulatory requirements, and maintains high standards of data quality and participant safety. Effective monitoring identifies potential issues early, allowing for timely interventions to address any concerns and maintain the integrity of the trial. Here are the key aspects of monitoring site performance:

Regular Site Visits:

- **On-site Monitoring:** Conducted by clinical research associates (CRAs) or monitors, on-site visits are critical for a thorough review of the trial processes, participant files, and data accuracy. These visits allow for direct observation of the site's operations, interaction with site staff, and verification of consent documentation, protocol adherence, and the handling of investigational products.

- **Remote Monitoring:** Leveraging technology to review site activities and data remotely has become increasingly prevalent, especially in the context of global challenges that limit travel. Remote monitoring includes the review of electronic medical records, data entries, and compliance documentation, providing an efficient and cost-effective way to oversee site performance.

Data Quality Checks:

- **Source Data Verification (SDV):** Monitors verify that data recorded in case report forms (CRFs) accurately reflect the source data (e.g., medical records, lab results). This process ensures the integrity and reliability of the trial data.

- **Query Resolution:** Discrepancies and inconsistencies identified during data review generate queries that the site must address and resolve promptly, ensuring the accuracy of the trial data.

Compliance and Adherence to Protocol:

- Monitoring assesses the site's adherence to the study protocol, including participant eligibility, treatment administration, and follow-up visits. Non-compliance or deviations from the protocol are documented and addressed to mitigate their impact on the study outcomes.

- Compliance with regulatory requirements and Good Clinical Practice (GCP) guidelines is also a focus of monitoring, ensuring that the trial upholds ethical standards and participant safety.

Safety Monitoring:

- Monitors review adverse event reports and safety data to ensure that all events are appropriately documented, reported, and managed according to the protocol and regulatory requirements.

- The monitoring process includes verifying that participants are informed of any new safety information that may affect their willingness to continue in the trial.

Performance Metrics and Continuous Improvement:

- Performance metrics, such as recruitment rates, retention rates, data entry timeliness, and query resolution times, are used to evaluate site performance objectively.

- Sites may receive feedback and training based on monitoring findings to address areas of concern and improve performance continuously.

Stakeholder Communication:

- Effective communication between site staff, monitors, and trial sponsors is crucial for addressing issues identified during monitoring visits. Regular updates, meetings, and reports ensure that all stakeholders are informed of the site's performance and any actions taken to resolve issues.

Monitoring site performance is a dynamic and ongoing process, requiring collaboration, communication, and a commitment to quality and ethical standards from all parties involved. By ensuring that sites operate efficiently, comply with protocols, and prioritize participant safety, monitoring plays a vital role in the successful execution and completion of clinical trials.

4.4 Exercise: 10 MCQs with Answers at the End

Multiple Choice Questions:

1. What is the primary goal of monitoring site performance in clinical trials?

- A) To increase the trial's budget

- B) To ensure adherence to the study protocol and regulatory requirements

- C) To promote the trial on social media

- D) To recruit more participants for the study

2. On-site monitoring visits are essential for:

- A) Reviewing financial statements of the site

- B) Direct observation of site operations and verification of data accuracy

- C) Redecorating the trial site

- D) Conducting local advertising campaigns

3. Remote monitoring in clinical trials allows for:

- A) Personal meetings with each participant

- B) Review of site activities and data remotely using technology

- C) Unlimited budget adjustments

- D) Physical inspection of site facilities

4. Source Data Verification (SDV) involves:

- A) Changing data to match expected outcomes

- B) Verifying that data recorded in case report forms accurately reflect source data

- C) Ignoring discrepancies in data

- D) Collecting new data to replace original findings

5. The resolution of data discrepancies and inconsistencies during monitoring generates:

- A) Promotional materials

- B) Financial incentives for sites

- C) Queries that the site must address and resolve

- D) Requests for additional funding

6. Compliance with Good Clinical Practice (GCP) guidelines during monitoring ensures:

- A) The trial's marketing strategy is effective

- B) Ethical standards and participant safety are upheld

- C) The site's social media presence is boosted

- D) Increased media coverage of the trial

7. The review of adverse event reports during monitoring is important for:

- A) Creating new advertising campaigns

- B) Ensuring all events are appropriately documented and managed

- C) Updating the trial's website

- D) Generating public relations materials

8. Performance metrics used in monitoring site performance may include:

   - A) Number of social media likes

   - B) Color scheme of the site's decor

   - C) Recruitment rates and data entry timeliness

   - D) Menu options in the site cafeteria

9. Continuous improvement in site performance is facilitated by:

   - A) Ignoring feedback from monitoring visits

   - B) Providing feedback and training based on monitoring findings

   - C) Reducing the frequency of monitoring visits

   - D) Limiting communication with site staff

10. Effective communication between site staff, monitors, and trial sponsors is crucial for:

   - A) Organizing social events

   - B) Addressing issues identified during monitoring visits

   - C) Discussing unrelated business opportunities

   - D) Planning vacation schedules

Answers:

1. B) To ensure adherence to the study protocol and regulatory requirements

2. B) Direct observation of site operations and verification of data accuracy

3. B) Review of site activities and data remotely using technology

4. B) Verifying that data recorded in case report forms accurately reflect source data

5. C) Queries that the site must address and resolve

6. B) Ethical standards and participant safety are upheld

7. B) Ensuring all events are appropriately documented and managed

8. C) Recruitment rates and data entry timeliness

9. B) Providing feedback and training based on monitoring findings

10. B) Addressing issues identified during monitoring visits

Chapter 5: Patient Recruitment and Retention

5.1 Strategies for Effective Recruitment

Effective patient recruitment is a critical aspect of clinical trial success, often determining the pace and feasibility of the entire study. Despite its importance, recruitment poses significant challenges, with many trials facing delays due to difficulties in enrolling enough participants. Employing strategic, thoughtful approaches to recruitment can enhance enrollment rates and ensure a diverse participant pool that reflects the study population. Here are key strategies for effective patient recruitment:

1. Clear Understanding of the Target Population:

- **Demographic Analysis:** Conduct a detailed analysis of the trial's target population, including age, gender, medical condition, and other relevant criteria, to understand where potential participants can be found and how best to approach them.

- **Inclusion/Exclusion Criteria Simplification:** Simplify inclusion and exclusion criteria without compromising the scientific integrity of the study to broaden the pool of eligible participants.

2. Multichannel Recruitment Campaigns:

- **Digital Platforms:** Use websites, social media, and online patient forums to raise awareness about the trial. Tailored ads and informational content can reach a wide audience quickly.

- **Traditional Media:** Newspapers, radio, and community bulletins can be effective, especially in reaching demographics less active online.

- **Patient Registries and Databases:** Utilize existing patient registries and healthcare databases to identify potential participants who meet the study criteria.

3. Community Engagement and Collaboration:

- **Partnerships with Healthcare Providers:** Collaborate with doctors, nurses, and other healthcare providers who can refer their patients to the trial. Providing them with clear information and benefits for their patients can encourage referrals.

- **Engagement with Patient Advocacy Groups:** Partner with advocacy groups related to the trial's focus area. These groups can help promote the trial to their members and provide valuable insights into patient needs and concerns.

- **Local Community Outreach:** Host informational sessions, health fairs, and workshops in community centers, libraries, and other local venues to engage directly with potential participants.

4. Patient-Centric Approaches:

- **Ease of Participation:** Minimize barriers to participation by offering flexible scheduling, transportation services, or virtual visits when possible.

- **Clear Communication:** Provide clear, jargon-free information about the trial's purpose, procedures, potential risks, and benefits to help potential participants make informed decisions.

- **Feedback Mechanisms:** Implement feedback mechanisms to learn from patients who choose not to participate or who drop out, using this information to improve recruitment strategies.

5. Financial and Non-Financial Incentives:

- **Compensation:** Offer fair compensation for participants' time and expenses, ensuring it is ethically appropriate and does not unduly influence participation.

- **Access to Care:** Highlight the potential benefits of participation, such as access to new treatments and close medical monitoring, which can be appealing to patients.

6. Continuous Monitoring and Adaptation:

- **Recruitment Metrics:** Track recruitment progress using metrics such as enrollment rates and participant diversity to identify and address bottlenecks quickly.

- **Adaptive Recruitment Strategies:** Be prepared to adapt recruitment strategies based on what is working or not, including trying new outreach methods or adjusting recruitment messages.

Effective patient recruitment requires a multifaceted approach that respects potential participants' needs and concerns while addressing the logistical and ethical complexities of enrolling patients in clinical trials. By employing diverse strategies and continuously evaluating their effectiveness, trial managers can enhance recruitment efforts, contributing to the timely and successful completion of clinical studies.

5.2 Ethical Considerations in Recruitment

The ethical recruitment of participants is foundational to the integrity of clinical research. Ensuring that recruitment practices are fair, transparent, and respectful of potential participants' rights and well-being is crucial. Here are key ethical considerations that must guide the recruitment process:

1. Informed Consent:

- **Comprehension:** Information provided to potential participants must be clear, accurate, and in a language and format that is understandable to them. It's crucial that participants comprehend the nature of the study, the procedures involved, potential risks and benefits, and their rights, including the right to withdraw at any time without penalty.

- **Voluntariness:** Participation in clinical trials must be voluntary, free from coercion or undue influence. Compensation should be carefully considered to ensure it does not coerce participation.

2. Respect for Privacy:

- **Confidentiality:** Protecting the privacy and confidentiality of potential and enrolled participants is paramount. Personal information must be securely handled and shared only with authorized personnel involved in the trial.

- **Sensitive Information:** Special care should be taken when dealing with sensitive or stigmatized conditions to avoid inadvertent disclosure that could harm participants.

3. Equitable Selection of Participants:

- **Avoidance of Exploitation:** Care must be taken to avoid exploiting vulnerable populations, including those with limited healthcare access, economic hardships, or diminished capacity to consent.

- **Inclusivity:** Recruitment strategies should aim for a diverse participant pool that accurately reflects the population affected by the condition under study. This includes ensuring gender, racial, and ethnic diversity to generalize the findings and understand differences in treatment effects.

4. Transparency and Honesty:

- **Accurate Representation:** All communications related to the trial, including advertisements, flyers, and verbal discussions, must accurately represent the study's purpose, procedures, and potential risks and benefits. Overselling the benefits or understating the risks can lead to mistrust and harm.

- **Disclosures:** Potential conflicts of interest or the sponsor's financial interests in the trial should be disclosed to participants to ensure transparency.

5. Regulatory and Ethical Approval:

- **Ethics Committee Review:** All recruitment materials and strategies must be reviewed and approved by an ethics committee or institutional review board (IRB) to ensure they meet ethical standards and regulatory requirements.

- **Adherence to Guidelines:** Recruitment practices should adhere to national and international guidelines on ethical conduct in human research, including the Declaration of Helsinki and Good Clinical Practice (GCP) guidelines.

6. Special Populations:

- **Additional Protections:** When recruiting children, pregnant women, or individuals with cognitive impairments, additional protections must be in place. This includes obtaining consent from guardians or legally authorized representatives and ensuring that participation poses minimal risk.

Ethical recruitment is not just a regulatory requirement but a moral imperative that upholds the dignity, rights, and welfare of participants. By embedding these ethical considerations into the recruitment process, researchers can foster trust, enhance participant engagement, and ensure the integrity and credibility of clinical trials.

5.3 Enhancing Participant Retention

Ensuring that participants remain engaged and enrolled in a clinical trial until its conclusion is just as crucial as recruiting them. High dropout rates can compromise the validity of the study results, lead to delays, and increase costs. Here are strategies to enhance participant retention:

1. Effective Communication:

- **Regular Updates:** Keep participants informed about the trial's progress and milestones. Transparency about any changes or updates in the study builds trust and a sense of involvement.

- **Open Channels:** Establish easy-to-use communication channels for participants to ask questions, express concerns, or report issues. Feeling heard and valued can significantly impact a participant's decision to stay in the study.

2. Participant Support and Engagement:

- **Orientation Sessions:** Provide comprehensive orientation sessions to set clear expectations and address any questions or concerns participants might have about the trial process.

- **Support Services:** Offer support services such as counseling, transportation, and reminders for appointments to reduce the burden of participation and address barriers that may lead to dropout.

3. Flexibility and Convenience:

- **Flexible Scheduling:** Accommodate participants' schedules as much as possible to make participation less disruptive to their daily lives.

- **Remote Participation Options:** Where feasible, use telehealth or mobile health technologies to allow participants to complete certain study procedures or follow-ups remotely.

4. Participant-Centric Approach:

- **Feedback Mechanisms:** Implement mechanisms for participants to provide feedback about their trial experience. Use this feedback to make continuous improvements in the trial process.

- **Cultural and Linguistic Sensitivity:** Ensure that trial materials and communication are culturally and linguistically appropriate, reflecting the diversity of the participant population.

5. Incentives and Compensation:

- **Ethical Incentives:** Offer fair compensation for time and expenses related to trial participation. Incentives should be ethically considered and should not coerce continued participation.

- **Acknowledgment:** Recognize and acknowledge the contribution of participants to the research, which can be a powerful motivator for continued engagement.

6. Education and Empowerment:

- **Informative Materials:** Provide educational materials about the condition being studied, the importance of the research, and how participants' contributions are making a difference.

- **Empowerment:** Engage participants as active partners in the research process, emphasizing the critical role they play in advancing medical knowledge.

7. Monitoring and Addressing Adverse Events:

- **Prompt Response:** Ensure that any reported adverse events are promptly addressed and communicated to participants. Knowing that their safety is a priority encourages trust and retention.

- **Support for Adverse Events:** Offer additional support and information to participants experiencing adverse events, helping them understand their options and the importance of reporting these events.

8. Continuity of Care:

- **Post-Trial Follow-up:** Offer post-trial follow-up care or information about where participants can receive ongoing treatment or support for their condition. This continuity of care demonstrates a commitment to their well-being beyond the study's end.

Enhancing participant retention requires a multifaceted approach focused on communication, support, flexibility, and recognition of participants' contributions. By implementing these strategies, researchers can minimize dropout rates, ensuring robust and reliable study outcomes.

5.4 Exercise: 10 MCQs with Answers at the End

Multiple Choice Questions:

1. What is a key factor in enhancing participant retention in clinical trials?

   - A) Reducing the number of site visits to a minimum

   - B) Effective communication and regular updates

   - C) Limiting participant access to trial information

   - D) Discouraging feedback from participants

2. How can flexibility and convenience contribute to participant retention?

   - A) By making trial participation more disruptive

   - B) By accommodating participants' schedules and offering remote participation options

   - C) By enforcing strict participation schedules

- D) By minimizing contact with participants

3. What role does offering support services play in participant retention?

- A) Decreases the likelihood of retention

- B) Increases participant burden

- C) Addresses barriers to participation and reduces dropout rates

- D) Has no impact on participant retention

4. Which approach is most effective in ensuring cultural and linguistic appropriateness in trial materials?

- A) Using technical jargon in all communications

- B) Ignoring cultural differences

- C) Tailoring materials to reflect the diversity of the participant population

- D) Providing materials in a single language only

5. What is the purpose of implementing feedback mechanisms for participants?

- A) To ignore participant suggestions and concerns

- B) To make continuous improvements in the trial process based on participant feedback

- C) To increase the complexity of trial participation

- D) To discourage participants from expressing their opinions

6. Why is offering fair compensation for time and expenses related to trial participation important?

   - A) To unduly influence participants to remain in the trial

   - B) To ensure ethical incentives and acknowledge participants' contributions

   - C) To minimize the value of participants' contributions

   - D) To create financial dependencies

7. How does empowering participants as active partners in research impact retention?

   - A) It decreases participants' interest in the trial

   - B) It makes participants feel undervalued

   - C) It emphasizes the critical role participants play in advancing medical knowledge

   - D) It reduces participants' understanding of the trial's importance

8. The prompt response to and support for adverse events is crucial for:

   - A) Discouraging participants from reporting negative experiences

   - B) Building trust and ensuring participants' safety is a priority

   - C) Overlooking the significance of adverse events

- D) Reducing the quality of data collected

9. Offering post-trial follow-up care or information demonstrates:

  - A) A lack of interest in participants' well-being after the trial

- B) A commitment to participants' well-being beyond the study's end

  - C) An effort to minimize trial costs

  - D) A strategy to limit participant engagement

10. Which strategy is least effective in enhancing participant retention?

  - A) Recognizing and acknowledging participants' contributions

  - B) Providing comprehensive orientation sessions

  - C) Limiting communication with participants

  - D) Offering educational materials about the condition being studied

Answers:

1. B) Effective communication and regular updates

2. B) By accommodating participants' schedules and offering remote participation options

3. C) Addresses barriers to participation and reduces dropout rates

4. C) Tailoring materials to reflect the diversity of the participant population

5. B) To make continuous improvements in the trial process based on participant feedback

6. B) To ensure ethical incentives and acknowledge participants' contributions

7. C) It emphasizes the critical role participants play in advancing medical knowledge

8. B) Building trust and ensuring participants' safety is a priority

9. B) A commitment to participants' well-being beyond the study's end

10. C) Limiting communication with participants

Chapter 6: Data Management and Integrity

6.1 Establishing Data Collection Methods

Establishing robust data collection methods is vital to the success of a clinical trial, ensuring the accuracy, reliability, and integrity of the data collected. These methods form the foundation upon which conclusions about the safety and efficacy of interventions are drawn. Effective data collection strategies are characterized by their ability to capture necessary information accurately and consistently across all participants and sites. Here are key considerations in establishing data collection methods for clinical trials:

1. Designing Case Report Forms (CRFs):

- **CRFs Creation:** Develop comprehensive CRFs, both paper-based and electronic (eCRFs), tailored to capture all trial-related data efficiently. These forms should be designed to minimize errors in data entry and ensure consistency across sites.

- **Pilot Testing:** Pilot test the CRFs in a small subset of the trial population or with trial staff to identify and rectify potential issues before full-scale implementation.

2. Selecting Data Collection Tools and Technologies:

- **Electronic Data Capture (EDC) Systems:** Utilize EDC systems for real-time data entry, storage, and management. These systems enhance data accuracy, facilitate remote monitoring, and streamline data analysis.

- **Mobile Health Technologies:** Consider using mobile health technologies, such as wearable devices and mobile apps, for continuous data collection, especially for parameters that require monitoring over time.

3. Training Staff on Data Collection Procedures:

- **Comprehensive Training:** Provide thorough training for all trial staff involved in data collection on the correct use of CRFs, EDC systems, and any other data collection tools to ensure high-quality data.

- **Certification and Recertification:** Implement certification processes to confirm staff competency in data collection methods, with periodic recertification to maintain high standards.

4. Standardizing Procedures Across Sites:

- **Standard Operating Procedures (SOPs):** Develop and disseminate SOPs for data collection across all trial sites to ensure uniformity in how data is collected, recorded, and entered.

- **Site Audits:** Conduct regular site audits to verify adherence to SOPs and identify any deviations or inconsistencies in data collection practices.

5. Ensuring Data Quality and Integrity:

- **Data Quality Checks:** Implement automated and manual data quality checks to identify missing, inconsistent, or outlying data, allowing for timely corrections.

- **Data Integrity Measures:** Employ measures to protect data integrity, including audit trails, data encryption, and access controls in EDC systems.

6. Incorporating Patient-Reported Outcomes:

- **Direct Data Collection:** When appropriate, include direct data collection from participants through patient-reported outcome measures (PROMs), using validated tools and scales to capture subjective outcomes related to quality of life, symptoms, and treatment satisfaction.

7. Regulatory Compliance and Documentation:

- **Compliance with Regulations:** Ensure that data collection methods comply with regulatory requirements, including those related to data protection and privacy (e.g., GDPR, HIPAA).

- **Documentation:** Maintain comprehensive documentation of all data collection processes, tools, and staff training records to support audit readiness and regulatory inspections.

By carefully establishing data collection methods, clinical trials can achieve the highest standards of data quality and integrity, underpinning the reliability of trial results and supporting sound conclusions about the interventions under study.

6.2 Ensuring Data Quality and Integrity

Ensuring data quality and integrity is paramount in clinical trials to maintain the trustworthiness of the results and ensure regulatory compliance. This involves implementing rigorous processes and controls throughout the data lifecycle, from collection through analysis. Here are key strategies to safeguard data quality and integrity in clinical research:

1. Data Validation and Verification:

- **Validation Rules:** Apply automated validation rules in data capture systems to check data entries for errors or inconsistencies in real time. This includes range checks, format checks, and logic checks to ensure data plausibility and consistency.

- **Source Data Verification (SDV):** For critical data points, perform SDV to compare the data recorded in the case report forms (CRFs) or electronic data capture (EDC) system against the original source data, such as medical records, laboratory reports, or other original documents.

2. Comprehensive Data Management Plan (DMP):

- **Establishing a DMP:** Develop a detailed DMP that outlines the data management processes, responsibilities, and standards to be adhered to throughout the trial. This plan should include procedures for data entry, coding, security, quality checks, backups, and archiving.

- **Review and Update:** Regularly review and update the DMP to reflect any changes in the trial or data management practices, ensuring ongoing relevance and compliance.

3. Regular Data Audits and Quality Checks:

- **Audits:** Conduct periodic audits of the data and data management processes to identify and rectify any issues that could impact data quality or integrity.

- **Quality Checks:** Implement routine data quality checks to identify missing, duplicate, or anomalous data entries for correction or clarification.

4. Training and Competency:

- **Staff Training:** Ensure all personnel involved in data management and entry are adequately trained and understand the importance of data quality and integrity. This includes training on the trial's protocols, data management systems, and privacy regulations.

- **Certification:** Consider certification or recertification processes for staff to demonstrate their competency in data management practices.

5. Data Security and Participant Privacy:

- **Access Controls:** Use robust access controls to restrict data access to authorized personnel only, protecting against unauthorized data viewing or manipulation.

- **Encryption and Secure Storage:** Employ data encryption during transmission and secure storage solutions, both physical and digital, to protect data from loss, theft, or corruption.

6. Documentation and Traceability:

- **Audit Trails:** Maintain comprehensive audit trails that log all data entries, changes, and accesses, including who made the change, what was changed, and when the change occurred. This facilitates traceability and accountability in data management.

- **Documentation:** Document all data management procedures, validations, quality checks, and audit findings to provide a clear trail for review and inspection.

7. Adherence to Regulations and Guidelines:

- **Regulatory Compliance:** Ensure data management practices comply with relevant regulatory requirements and industry standards, including Good Clinical Practice (GCP) and data protection laws (e.g., GDPR, HIPAA).

- **Guideline Alignment:** Align data management processes with best practices and guidelines from regulatory authorities and professional organizations to ensure the highest standards of data quality and integrity.

Ensuring data quality and integrity is a continuous effort that requires the collaboration of all trial stakeholders. By implementing these strategies, researchers can safeguard the credibility of their findings, protect participant data, and contribute valuable knowledge to the scientific community.

6.3 Data Analysis and Interpretation

Data analysis and interpretation are critical stages in clinical trials, transforming raw data into meaningful insights that can guide medical decisions and policy. This phase requires meticulous planning, execution, and a clear understanding of statistical principles to ensure the validity and reliability of the conclusions drawn. Here are essential aspects of data analysis and interpretation in clinical research:

1. Statistical Analysis Plan (SAP):

- **Pre-specification:** Develop a detailed SAP before initiating the data analysis. The SAP should outline the statistical methods to be used, the primary and secondary endpoints, subgroup analyses, handling of missing data, and any interim analyses planned.

- **Flexibility and Rigor:** While the SAP should allow some flexibility to explore unexpected findings, it must also adhere to rigorous standards to prevent data dredging and ensure that the results are statistically valid and reproducible.

2. Handling of Missing Data:

- **Assessment:** Evaluate the extent and pattern of missing data, considering how it may impact the study's outcomes. The reasons for missing data should be explored, as they can provide insights into potential biases.

- **Strategies:** Apply appropriate statistical methods to handle missing data, such as multiple imputation or sensitivity analyses, to minimize bias and ensure the robustness of the study conclusions.

3. Interim Analyses and Stopping Rules:

- **Interim Analyses:** Plan for interim analyses to assess the data at predetermined points during the trial. This can help in making decisions about continuing, modifying, or stopping the trial early for efficacy, futility, or safety reasons.

- **Stopping Rules:** Clearly define the criteria for prematurely ending the trial in the SAP, ensuring that these decisions are based on solid statistical evidence and ethical considerations.

4. Data Interpretation:

- **Contextual Analysis:** Interpret the data within the context of the study's objectives, the existing body of scientific evidence, and clinical relevance. Avoid overinterpretation of statistically significant findings without considering their practical significance.

- **Subgroup Analyses:** Conduct subgroup analyses with caution, recognizing that findings may be due to chance, especially if the analyses were not pre-specified. Subgroup analyses should be hypothesis-generating rather than conclusive.

5. Transparency and Reproducibility:

- **Reporting Standards:** Adhere to established reporting standards, such as CONSORT for randomized trials, to ensure transparency in how the study was conducted and analyzed.

- **Data Sharing:** Consider sharing de-identified trial data with the broader scientific community to enable independent verification of the results and further research, in accordance with ethical guidelines and participant consent.

6. Communication of Results:

- **Clear Presentation:** Present the results in a clear, concise manner, using appropriate tables, figures, and statistical measures to convey the findings effectively.

- **Discussion of Limitations:** Discuss the limitations of the analysis openly, including potential biases, uncertainties, and the generalizability of the findings.

7. Ethical Considerations:

- **Beneficence and Non-Maleficence:** Ensure that the interpretation and dissemination of results do no harm and contribute positively to scientific knowledge and patient care.

- **Participant Welfare:** Consider the implications of the study findings for the participants, especially if the results have direct clinical relevance.

Effective data analysis and interpretation are pivotal in deriving meaningful conclusions from clinical trials, guiding future research, and informing clinical practice. By adhering to rigorous statistical and ethical standards, researchers can ensure the integrity and utility of their findings.

6.4 Exercise: 10 MCQs with Answers at the End

Multiple Choice Questions:

1. What is the purpose of a Statistical Analysis Plan (SAP) in clinical trials?

   - A) To guide the marketing strategy for the trial

   - B) To outline the statistical methods and analyses to be used

   - C) To list the participants' names and data

- D) To describe the trial's budget in detail

2. Which strategy is essential for handling missing data in clinical trials?

   - A) Ignoring all missing data as irrelevant

   - B) Using the last observation carried forward (LOCF) method indiscriminately

   - C) Applying appropriate statistical methods, such as multiple imputation

   - D) Deleting any cases with missing data

3. The primary reason for conducting interim analyses in a clinical trial is to:

   - A) Increase the trial duration

   - B) Assess data at predetermined points for critical decisions

   - C) Postpone data analysis until the end of the trial

   - D) Avoid reporting the results

4. In data interpretation, the contextual analysis involves:

   - A) Ignoring the study's objectives

   - B) Interpreting data without considering clinical relevance

   - C) Considering the existing body of scientific evidence and clinical relevance

   - D) Focusing solely on statistically significant results

5. Subgroup analyses in clinical trials should be:

- A) The primary method for drawing conclusions

- B) Conducted without pre-specification

- C) Viewed as hypothesis-generating rather than conclusive

- D) Used to prove causality

6. Which of the following is true about the transparency and reproducibility of trial data?

- A) Keeping the data and methods confidential is best practice

- B) Sharing de-identified trial data promotes independent verification

- C) Using proprietary methods that cannot be disclosed improves credibility

- D) Results should be shared only with those who funded the trial

7. The CONSORT guidelines are designed to:

- A) Decrease the transparency of clinical trials

- B) Provide a standard for reporting randomized controlled trials

- C) Complicate the publication process

- D) Limit the sharing of trial results

8. Ethical considerations in data analysis and interpretation include:

 - A) Benefiting only the research team

 - B) Prioritizing statistical significance over clinical relevance

 - C) Ensuring participant welfare and contributing positively to scientific knowledge

 - D) Ignoring the potential harm from misinterpretation of results

9. Why is it important to discuss the limitations of the analysis openly?

 - A) To undermine the study's findings

- B) To highlight potential biases, uncertainties, and generalizability issues

 - C) To discourage further research

 - D) To focus solely on the strengths of the study

10. Effective communication of results involves:

 - A) Presenting data in a complex and technical manner

 - B) Clear presentation using appropriate statistical measures

 - C) Excluding tables and figures for simplicity

 - D) Avoiding the discussion of study limitations

Answers:

1. B) To outline the statistical methods and analyses to be used

2. C) Applying appropriate statistical methods, such as multiple imputation

3. B) Assess data at predetermined points for critical decisions

4. C) Considering the existing body of scientific evidence and clinical relevance

5. C) Viewed as hypothesis-generating rather than conclusive

6. B) Sharing de-identified trial data promotes independent verification

7. B) Provide a standard for reporting randomized controlled trials

8. C) Ensuring participant welfare and contributing positively to scientific knowledge

9. B) To highlight potential biases, uncertainties, and generalizability issues

10. B) Clear presentation using appropriate statistical measures

Chapter 7: Regulatory Compliance and Audits

7.1 Understanding Regulatory Requirements

Regulatory compliance is a cornerstone of clinical trial management, ensuring that studies are conducted ethically, safely, and in accordance with established standards. Understanding and adhering to regulatory requirements is crucial for protecting participant welfare, ensuring data integrity, and facilitating the acceptance and publication of study results. Here's an overview of key regulatory aspects in clinical research:

1. Good Clinical Practice (GCP):

- **International Standard:** GCP is an international ethical and scientific quality standard for designing, conducting, recording, and reporting trials that involve the participation of human subjects. Compliance with GCP ensures that the rights, safety, and well-being of trial participants are protected, and that the trial data are credible.

- **ICH-GCP Guidelines:** The International Council for Harmonisation of Technical Requirements for Pharmaceuticals for Human Use (ICH) provides guidelines that are widely accepted as the benchmark for GCP. These guidelines cover aspects such as investigator qualifications, trial design, conduct, record-keeping, and reporting.

2. Regulatory Authorities:

- **Local and National Regulations:** Clinical trials are subject to regulatory oversight by national health authorities, such as the Food and Drug Administration (FDA) in the United States, the European Medicines Agency (EMA) in the European Union, and other regulatory bodies worldwide. These authorities enforce regulations that govern clinical trials in their jurisdictions, including trial approval processes, participant consent, and reporting of adverse events.

- **Ethics Committees/Institutional Review Boards (IRBs):** Ethics committees or IRBs review and approve the ethical aspects of clinical trials, ensuring that studies comply with ethical standards and regulatory requirements. Approval from an ethics committee or IRB is required before a trial can commence.

3. Informed Consent:

- **Essential Process:** Informed consent is a fundamental ethical and legal requirement for conducting clinical trials. It involves providing potential participants with all necessary information about the trial, including its purpose, procedures, risks, benefits, and the right to withdraw at any time, and obtaining their voluntary agreement to participate.

- **Documentation:** The informed consent process must be documented, typically through a signed consent form, which must be approved by the ethics committee or IRB.

4. Data Protection and Privacy:

- **Confidentiality of Participant Information:** Regulations such as the General Data Protection Regulation (GDPR) in the European Union and the Health Insurance Portability and Accountability Act (HIPAA) in the United States set standards for the protection of personal and health information of trial participants.

- **Data Security Measures:** Clinical trials must implement measures to safeguard participant data, including secure data storage, controlled access, and ensuring data confidentiality during and after the trial.

5. Adverse Event Reporting:

- **Safety Monitoring:** Regulatory requirements mandate the monitoring and reporting of adverse events and other safety information to regulatory authorities, ethics committees, and sponsors. This is crucial for ongoing assessment of the intervention's risk-benefit ratio.

6. Trial Registration and Results Reporting:

- **Public Disclosure:** Many jurisdictions require clinical trials to be registered in public databases before initiation, and results to be reported upon completion, enhancing transparency and accountability in research.

Understanding and complying with these regulatory requirements is not only a legal obligation but also a commitment to ethical conduct and scientific integrity. Navigating the regulatory landscape requires continuous vigilance, as regulations and guidelines can evolve in response to new scientific knowledge and societal expectations.

7.2 Preparing for Audits and Inspections

Preparing for audits and inspections is a critical aspect of clinical trial management, ensuring compliance with regulatory requirements and maintaining the integrity of the trial. These evaluations can be conducted by regulatory authorities, sponsors, or independent audit organizations to verify adherence to Good Clinical Practice (GCP) guidelines, regulatory obligations, and the study protocol. Effective preparation can help identify and address potential issues proactively, facilitating a smooth audit or inspection process. Here are key strategies for preparing for audits and inspections in clinical trials:

1. Establish a Culture of Compliance:

- **Continuous Compliance:** Foster an environment where compliance with GCP and regulatory requirements is part of daily operations, not just a focus during audits.

- **Education and Training:** Regularly train staff on regulatory requirements, the importance of documentation, and the principles of GCP to ensure everyone understands their roles and responsibilities.

2. Conduct Internal Audits:

- **Proactive Assessments:** Implement a schedule for regular internal audits to assess the trial's compliance status and identify areas for improvement.

- **Corrective Action Plans:** Develop and execute corrective action plans for any non-compliance issues identified during internal audits, documenting the steps taken to resolve the issues.

3. Maintain Accurate and Complete Documentation:

- **Trial Master File (TMF):** Ensure the Trial Master File is up-to-date and organized, containing all essential documents that demonstrate the trial's compliance with GCP and regulatory requirements.

- **Document Management:** Regularly review and update documentation practices to ensure all study-related records are accurate, complete, and easily accessible for auditors.

4. Prepare Staff for the Audit Process:

- **Roles and Responsibilities:** Clearly define and communicate the roles and responsibilities of staff members during an audit or inspection.

- **Mock Audits:** Conduct mock audits or inspection drills to familiarize staff with the audit process and reduce anxiety, improving their performance during actual audits.

5. Review Regulatory Guidelines and Updates:

- **Stay Informed:** Regularly review regulatory guidelines and updates from relevant authorities (e.g., FDA, EMA) to ensure the trial remains compliant with current standards.

- **Regulatory Consultations:** Seek clarification or guidance from regulatory authorities if there are uncertainties about compliance requirements.

6. Develop an Audit Plan:

- **Logistics and Coordination:** Prepare a detailed plan outlining the logistics of the audit, including the schedule, location, access to documents, and personnel involved.

- **Communication:** Establish clear lines of communication with the auditing body, providing necessary information and coordinating logistics prior to the audit.

7. Manage the Audit Process:

- **Point of Contact:** Designate a knowledgeable and experienced staff member as the primary point of contact for auditors to facilitate efficient communication and information exchange.

- **Address Findings Promptly:** Respond to any findings or observations made during the audit promptly and thoroughly, with a clear plan for corrective and preventive actions.

Preparing for audits and inspections requires a proactive and systematic approach to ensure that clinical trials are conducted in compliance with regulatory standards and GCP guidelines. By adopting these strategies, trial sponsors and investigators can minimize compliance risks, address potential issues before they become problematic, and demonstrate their commitment to conducting ethical and reliable clinical research.

7.3 Handling Non-compliance Issues

Non-compliance issues in clinical trials can range from minor procedural deviations to significant violations of regulatory requirements or Good Clinical Practice (GCP) guidelines. Effective handling of these issues is crucial to maintain the integrity of the trial, ensure participant safety, and uphold ethical standards. Here are strategies for effectively addressing non-compliance issues in clinical trials:

1. Immediate Assessment:

- **Identify and Document:** Quickly identify and document the non-compliance issue, including when and how it occurred, and the parties involved.

- **Assess Severity:** Assess the severity and potential impact of the non-compliance on the trial's integrity, participant safety, and data validity.

2. Notification and Reporting:

- **Internal Notification:** Immediately inform trial oversight bodies, such as the principal investigator, the trial sponsor, and the institutional review board (IRB) or ethics committee.

- **Regulatory Reporting:** Report the non-compliance to regulatory authorities if required by law or regulation, following the specified timelines and procedures.

3. Root Cause Analysis:

- **Investigate Cause:** Conduct a thorough investigation to determine the root cause(s) of the non-compliance, whether it be human error, lack of training, procedural ambiguities, or system failures.

- **Engage Stakeholders:** Involve relevant stakeholders in the investigation process, including study staff, participants (if applicable), and external experts, to ensure a comprehensive understanding of the issue.

4. Corrective and Preventive Actions (CAPA):

- **Develop a CAPA Plan:** Develop a corrective and preventive action plan to address the non-compliance issue and prevent its recurrence. This may include retraining staff, revising protocols or procedures, and enhancing monitoring and oversight mechanisms.

- **Implementation and Monitoring:** Implement the CAPA plan promptly and monitor its effectiveness over time, making adjustments as necessary to ensure the issue is fully resolved.

5. Documentation and Communication:

- **Comprehensive Documentation:** Document all steps taken to address the non-compliance issue, including the initial assessment, investigation findings, CAPA plan, and monitoring efforts.

- **Transparent Communication:** Communicate openly with all relevant parties, including trial participants, regulatory authorities, and the public (if appropriate), about the non-compliance issue and the steps taken to address it, maintaining transparency and trust.

6. Training and Education:

- **Lessons Learned:** Use the non-compliance issue as a learning opportunity to strengthen the trial's compliance and oversight. Share lessons learned with trial staff and incorporate them into training and education programs.

- **Ongoing Compliance Training:** Enhance ongoing compliance training for trial staff to prevent future non-compliance issues, focusing on areas identified as weaknesses in the current incident.

7. Review and Update Trial Procedures:

- **Procedure Updates:** Review and, if necessary, update trial procedures, SOPs, and documentation practices based on the lessons learned from handling the non-compliance issue to strengthen trial governance and compliance.

Effectively handling non-compliance issues requires prompt action, thorough investigation, and transparent communication. By adopting a systematic approach to addressing these issues, clinical trial stakeholders can safeguard the trial's integrity, ensure participant safety, and maintain regulatory compliance.

7.4 Exercise: 10 MCQs with Answers at the End

Multiple Choice Questions:

1. What is the first step in handling non-compliance issues in clinical trials?

   - A) Ignoring the issue to avoid penalties

   - B) Immediately assessing and documenting the issue

   - C) Reporting the issue to the media

   - D) Dismissing involved staff members

2. To whom should non-compliance issues be immediately reported internally?

   - A) Only to the study sponsor

   - B) To the principal investigator, trial sponsor, and IRB/ethics committee

   - C) To the participants

   - D) To competing research groups

3. A thorough investigation of non-compliance issues aims to:

   - A) Assign blame to specific individuals

   - B) Determine the root cause(s) of the issue

- C) Cover up the issue as quickly as possible

- D) Penalize the research institution

4. Corrective and Preventive Actions (CAPA) plans are developed to:

- A) Increase the trial budget

- B) Address the issue and prevent its recurrence

- C) Complicate trial procedures

- D) Shorten the trial duration

5. When should regulatory authorities be notified of non-compliance?

- A) After the trial concludes

- B) Only if the media finds out

- C) If required by law or regulation, following specified timelines

- D) Never, to avoid fines

6. The effectiveness of a CAPA plan should be:

- A) Assumed without verification

- B) Monitored over time and adjusted as necessary

- C) Evaluated once without further follow-up

- D) Ignored after implementation

7. Which of the following is an essential aspect of handling non-compliance?

   - A) Ensuring no documentation is kept

   - B) Comprehensive documentation of all steps taken

   - C) Limiting communication about the issue

   - D) Avoiding analysis of the issue's root cause

8. Lessons learned from non-compliance issues should be:

   - A) Hidden from new staff members

   - B) Used as a basis for enhancing training and education programs

   - C) Considered irrelevant for future trials

   - D) Used to criticize the trial team

9. The purpose of reviewing and updating trial procedures after handling non-compliance is to:

   - A) Simplify documentation requirements

   - B) Strengthen trial governance and compliance

   - C) Reduce the number of staff involved in the trial

   - D) Decrease transparency in trial operations

10. Why is transparent communication important in handling non-compliance issues?

   - A) To confuse trial participants and sponsors

   - B) To maintain transparency and trust among all relevant parties

   - C) To make the trial appear more successful

   - D) To minimize the importance of compliance

Answers:

1. B) Immediately assessing and documenting the issue

2. B) To the principal investigator, trial sponsor, and IRB/ethics committee

3. B) Determine the root cause(s) of the issue

4. B) Address the issue and prevent its recurrence

5. C) If required by law or regulation, following specified timelines

6. B) Monitored over time and adjusted as necessary

7. B) Comprehensive documentation of all steps taken

8. B) Used as a basis for enhancing training and education programs

9. B) Strengthen trial governance and compliance

10. B) To maintain transparency and trust among all relevant parties

Chapter 8: Risk Management

8.1 Identifying and Assessing Risks

Risk management is a crucial component of clinical trial management, aimed at identifying, assessing, and mitigating potential risks that could impact the trial's success, participant safety, data integrity, and compliance with regulatory requirements. The process of identifying and assessing risks involves a systematic approach to foreseeing potential problems and planning for them in advance. Here's how this critical phase is approached:

1. Establishing a Risk Management Plan:

- **Initial Planning:** Develop a risk management plan at the beginning of the trial, incorporating input from all stakeholders, including investigators, sponsors, regulatory experts, and patient representatives.

- **Scope and Objectives:** Clearly define the scope of the risk management activities and the objectives, including protecting participant safety, ensuring data quality, and maintaining regulatory compliance.

2. Risk Identification:

- **Brainstorming and Expert Consultation:** Use brainstorming sessions and consult with subject matter experts to identify potential risks across all aspects of the trial, from study design to data collection and reporting.

- **Review of Similar Trials:** Examine the challenges and issues encountered in similar previous trials as a source of information for potential risks.

- **Checklists and Templates:** Utilize checklists and risk assessment templates designed for clinical trials to ensure a comprehensive identification of risks.

3. Risk Categorization:

- **Categories:** Classify identified risks into categories such as operational, strategic, financial, regulatory, and ethical risks to streamline the assessment and mitigation processes.

- **Sources and Triggers:** Identify the sources of each risk and possible triggers that could cause the risk to materialize, facilitating targeted risk mitigation strategies.

4. Risk Assessment:

- **Likelihood and Impact:** Evaluate each identified risk for its likelihood of occurrence and potential impact on the trial. This assessment helps prioritize risks based on their severity.

- **Risk Matrix:** Use a risk matrix to visually map the risks according to their likelihood and impact, aiding in the prioritization and allocation of resources for risk mitigation.

5. Documentation:

- **Risk Register:** Maintain a risk register that documents all identified risks, their assessment, and planned mitigation strategies. The risk register should be a living document, updated throughout the trial as new risks emerge or existing risks evolve.

6. Continuous Monitoring:

- **Regular Reviews:** Conduct regular reviews of the risk management plan and the risk register to assess the effectiveness of mitigation strategies and to identify new risks as the trial progresses.

- **Adaptive Management:** Be prepared to adapt risk mitigation strategies based on the outcomes of monitoring activities and changes in the trial or external environment.

Identifying and assessing risks in clinical trials is an ongoing process that requires vigilance, flexibility, and a proactive approach. By systematically identifying potential risks and assessing their likelihood and impact, trial managers can develop effective strategies to mitigate these risks, thereby safeguarding the trial's objectives, participant safety, and data integrity.

8.2 Implementing Risk Mitigation Strategies

Once risks in a clinical trial have been identified and assessed, the next critical step is the implementation of risk mitigation strategies. These strategies are designed to either prevent the occurrence of risks or minimize their impact should they materialize. Effective risk mitigation requires careful planning, resource allocation, and ongoing monitoring to ensure the strategies are effective. Here are essential steps and considerations in implementing risk mitigation strategies for clinical trials:

1. Prioritization of Risks:

- **Focus on High-Impact Risks:** Prioritize risks based on their potential impact on participant safety, trial integrity, and compliance. Allocate resources and efforts to mitigate high-priority risks first.

- **Balancing Act:** While focusing on high-impact risks, do not completely ignore lower-priority risks. Implement scalable and cost-effective strategies to manage these risks adequately.

2. Development of Mitigation Plans:

- **Specific Strategies for Each Risk:** Develop detailed mitigation plans for each identified risk, outlining specific actions, responsible parties, timelines, and required resources.

- **Preventive and Contingency Measures:** Include both preventive measures to avoid the risk and contingency measures to manage the risk if it occurs.

3. Engagement of Stakeholders:

- **Collaboration:** Engage all relevant stakeholders, including the trial team, sponsors, regulatory authorities, and participants, in the development and implementation of risk mitigation strategies.

- **Communication Plan:** Develop a communication plan to ensure all stakeholders are informed about the risk mitigation strategies and their roles in implementing these strategies.

4. Training and Education:

- **Staff Training:** Provide comprehensive training for trial staff on the risk mitigation strategies, emphasizing the importance of adherence to protocols and procedures designed to minimize risks.

- **Participant Education:** Educate participants about potential risks and the measures taken to protect them, enhancing their understanding and cooperation.

5. Integration with Trial Processes:

- **Seamless Integration:** Integrate risk mitigation strategies into existing trial processes and workflows to ensure they do not disrupt trial activities or add unnecessary complexity.

- **Standard Operating Procedures (SOPs):** Update or develop SOPs to include risk mitigation strategies, ensuring consistency and adherence across all trial sites.

6. Monitoring and Adjustment:

- **Ongoing Monitoring:** Continuously monitor the effectiveness of risk mitigation strategies through regular assessments, audits, and reviews.

- **Flexibility to Adjust:** Be prepared to adjust strategies as needed based on monitoring outcomes, new information, or changes in the trial or external environment.

7. Documentation and Reporting:

- **Documenting Actions:** Keep detailed records of all risk mitigation activities, including decisions made, actions taken, and outcomes achieved.

- **Regulatory Reporting:** Report significant risk mitigation actions and their outcomes to regulatory authorities as required.

8. Review and Learning:

- **Post-Trial Review:** After the trial concludes, review the effectiveness of the risk mitigation strategies to identify lessons learned and best practices.

- **Knowledge Sharing:** Share these insights within the organization and with the broader research community to improve risk management in future trials.

Implementing risk mitigation strategies in clinical trials is a dynamic process that requires proactive planning, stakeholder engagement, and the flexibility to adapt to changing circumstances. By effectively managing risks, trial managers can protect participants, ensure the integrity of trial data, and comply with regulatory requirements, thereby contributing to the success of the trial and the advancement of medical science.

8.3 Monitoring and Reporting Risks

Monitoring and reporting risks are pivotal components of the risk management process in clinical trials. Continuous oversight is crucial for detecting new risks, evaluating the effectiveness of mitigation strategies, and ensuring prompt communication of risk-related information to all stakeholders. This proactive approach helps in maintaining the integrity of the trial, safeguarding participant safety, and adhering to regulatory requirements. Here's how to effectively manage the monitoring and reporting of risks in clinical trials:

1. Continuous Risk Monitoring:

- **Ongoing Surveillance:** Implement an ongoing surveillance system to monitor identified risks and detect new risks throughout the trial's duration. This includes monitoring data trends, adverse events, and compliance indicators.

- **Risk Indicators:** Utilize predefined risk indicators or metrics to objectively assess the status of specific risks. These could include metrics related to participant recruitment, protocol deviations, data quality issues, or safety signals.

2. Regular Risk Assessments:

- **Scheduled Reviews:** Conduct regular risk assessment meetings with the trial management team to review the status of existing risks, evaluate the emergence of new risks, and assess the effectiveness of mitigation strategies.

- **Dynamic Risk Management:** Be prepared to update the risk management plan and mitigation strategies based on the findings from these assessments, adopting a dynamic approach to risk management.

3. Effective Communication Channels:

- **Stakeholder Engagement:** Ensure effective communication channels are in place for reporting risk information to all relevant stakeholders, including trial sponsors, regulatory authorities, ethics committees, and participants.

- **Clear Reporting Protocols:** Establish clear protocols for the escalation and reporting of significant risk findings or incidents. This includes determining thresholds for reporting, responsible parties for communication, and required timelines.

4. Documentation and Record-Keeping:

- **Risk Management Documentation:** Maintain comprehensive documentation of all risk monitoring activities, including risk assessments, changes to risk status, and actions taken in response to risk findings.

- **Audit Trail:** Ensure that an audit trail is kept for all risk-related decisions and communications, providing a transparent record for future reference or regulatory inspections.

5. Training and Awareness:

- **Staff Training:** Regularly train trial staff on risk monitoring procedures and the importance of risk awareness. Empower staff to recognize and report potential risks promptly.

- **Participant Information:** Keep trial participants informed about potential risks and any changes to the trial that may affect them, maintaining trust and transparency.

6. Regulatory and Ethical Compliance:

- **Compliance with Guidelines:** Ensure that risk monitoring and reporting activities comply with relevant regulatory guidelines and ethical standards, such as Good Clinical Practice (GCP).

- **Reporting to Authorities:** Adhere to requirements for reporting significant risks, especially those affecting participant safety, to regulatory authorities and ethics committees within specified timelines.

7. Utilizing Technology and Tools:

- **Risk Management Tools:** Utilize specialized software or tools designed for risk monitoring in clinical trials. These tools can help in tracking risk indicators, facilitating risk assessments, and streamlining communication.

- **Data Analytics:** Apply data analytics techniques to analyze trial data for emerging trends or patterns that may indicate potential risks.

Monitoring and reporting risks in clinical trials is a dynamic and integral part of risk management, requiring constant vigilance, effective communication, and a commitment to transparency and compliance. By systematically overseeing risks, trial managers can proactively address challenges, ensuring the trial remains on track to achieve its objectives while protecting the well-being of participants.

8.4 Exercise: 10 MCQs with Answers at the End

Multiple Choice Questions:

1. What is the primary goal of continuous risk monitoring in clinical trials?

   - A) To increase trial costs unnecessarily

   - B) To detect new risks and evaluate the effectiveness of mitigation strategies

   - C) To reduce communication with stakeholders

   - D) To ignore emerging risks until they become critical

2. Which method is used to objectively assess the status of specific risks in a trial?

   - A) Ignoring data trends and participant feedback

   - B) Utilizing predefined risk indicators or metrics

   - C) Making decisions based on assumptions without data

   - D) Relying solely on external audits

3. Regular risk assessments should lead to what action?

   - A) Discontinuing the trial immediately

   - B) No action, regardless of findings

- C) Updating the risk management plan and mitigation strategies as needed

   - D) Decreasing communication about risks

4. Effective communication channels for reporting risk information are essential for engaging which of the following stakeholders?

   - A) Only the trial participants

   - B) Only the regulatory authorities

   - C) Only the trial sponsors

   - D) All relevant stakeholders, including sponsors, regulatory authorities, ethics committees, and participants

5. What is crucial for maintaining a transparent record of risk-related decisions and communications?

   - A) Avoiding documentation of discussions and actions

   - B) Maintaining comprehensive documentation and an audit trail

   - C) Deleting records periodically to save space

   - D) Keeping records confidential from regulatory authorities

6. Regular training on risk monitoring procedures is important for which group of individuals?

- A) Trial participants only

- B) Regulatory authorities only

- C) Trial management staff

- D) External stakeholders only

7. Compliance with which guidelines is essential for risk monitoring and reporting activities?

- A) Food service guidelines

- B) Good Clinical Practice (GCP) and relevant regulatory guidelines

- C) Interior design standards

- D) Recreational activity guidelines

8. Reporting significant risks to regulatory authorities and ethics committees must be done within what framework?

- A) Specified timelines

- B) At the conclusion of the trial

- C) At the discretion of the trial staff

- D) Only if directly asked by an authority

9. Utilizing specialized software or tools for risk monitoring in clinical trials helps in:

- A) Reducing transparency and accountability

- B) Tracking risk indicators and facilitating risk assessments

- C) Ignoring participant safety concerns

- D) Increasing the complexity of trial management unnecessarily

10. Data analytics can be applied in risk monitoring to:

- A) Disregard data trends and patterns

- B) Analyze trial data for emerging trends or patterns indicating potential risks

- C) Reduce the amount of data collected during the trial

- D) Focus solely on past data without considering current or future implications

Answers:

1. B) To detect new risks and evaluate the effectiveness of mitigation strategies

2. B) Utilizing predefined risk indicators or metrics

3. C) Updating the risk management plan and mitigation strategies as needed

4. D) All relevant stakeholders, including sponsors, regulatory authorities, ethics committees, and participants

5. B) Maintaining comprehensive documentation and an audit trail

6. C) Trial management staff

7. B) Good Clinical Practice (GCP) and relevant regulatory guidelines

8. A) Specified timelines

9. B) Tracking risk indicators and facilitating risk assessments

10. B) Analyze trial data for emerging trends or patterns indicating potential risks

Chapter 9: Quality Assurance

9.1 Principles of Quality Assurance in Clinical Trials

Quality assurance (QA) in clinical trials is the systematic process of ensuring that the conduct of the trial and the generation, documentation, and reporting of data adhere to established standards, regulations, and ethical principles. QA is crucial for safeguarding the integrity of the trial data, ensuring participant safety, and maintaining public trust in the research process. The following principles are foundational to implementing effective quality assurance in clinical trials:

1. Adherence to Good Clinical Practice (GCP):

- **Global Standard:** GCP is an international ethical and scientific quality standard for designing, conducting, monitoring, recording, auditing, analyzing, and reporting trials. Adherence to GCP ensures that the rights, safety, and well-being of trial participants are protected while also providing assurance of the credibility and reliability of trial data.

- **Regulatory Compliance:** QA processes must ensure that the trial complies with all relevant local, national, and international regulations and guidelines governing clinical research.

2. Systematic Approach to Quality Management:

- **Quality Planning:** Develop a quality management plan that outlines the QA strategies, objectives, procedures, and responsibilities throughout the trial lifecycle, from protocol development to final reporting.

- **Risk-based Approach:** Implement a risk-based QA approach that prioritizes resources and efforts based on the potential impact of identified risks on participant safety and data integrity.

3. Continuous Monitoring and Improvement:

- **Proactive Monitoring:** Conduct ongoing monitoring of trial processes and data to promptly identify and address issues that could compromise quality. This includes both on-site and remote monitoring activities.

- **Corrective and Preventive Actions (CAPA):** Establish mechanisms for identifying, documenting, and addressing non-compliance or deviations from the protocol or SOPs. Implement corrective actions to resolve current issues and preventive actions to avoid future occurrences.

4. Training and Competency:

- **Staff Qualifications:** Ensure that all personnel involved in the trial, including investigators, research staff, and monitors, are appropriately qualified, trained, and competent to perform their assigned tasks.

- **Continuous Education:** Provide ongoing training and education to maintain and update the knowledge and skills of the trial team, reinforcing the importance of quality in every aspect of the trial.

5. Documentation and Record-keeping:

- **Accurate and Complete Documentation:** Maintain comprehensive and accurate documentation of all trial activities, decisions, and findings. This documentation serves as the basis for evaluating the conduct of the trial and the quality of the data collected.

- **Audit Trail:** Implement an effective system for creating and maintaining an audit trail for all trial-related documents and data, facilitating traceability and accountability.

6. Independent Audits and Inspections:

- **Regular Audits:** Schedule regular independent audits to objectively assess compliance with the protocol, SOPs, GCP, and regulatory requirements. Audits help identify areas for improvement and reinforce the culture of quality.

- **Regulatory Inspections:** Prepare for and cooperate with regulatory inspections, using them as opportunities to demonstrate the trial's commitment to quality and regulatory compliance.

7. Stakeholder Engagement:

- **Collaboration:** Engage all stakeholders, including sponsors, regulatory authorities, ethics committees, and participants, in the quality management process. Open communication and collaboration enhance the effectiveness of QA efforts.

Quality assurance in clinical trials is not just a regulatory requirement but a commitment to ethical research practices, participant safety, and the generation of reliable data. By embedding these principles into every stage of the trial, researchers can achieve the highest standards of quality and integrity.

9.2 Developing a Quality Assurance Plan

A Quality Assurance (QA) Plan is a comprehensive document that outlines the strategies, procedures, and measures in place to ensure that a clinical trial is conducted in compliance with Good Clinical Practice (GCP), regulatory requirements, and the study protocol. The plan is pivotal in safeguarding the integrity of the trial data and ensuring participant safety. Here's a guide to developing an effective QA Plan for clinical trials:

1. Define Quality Objectives:

- **Clear Objectives:** Start by defining clear, measurable quality objectives aligned with GCP standards, regulatory requirements, and the specific goals of the clinical trial. Objectives may include ensuring data accuracy, participant safety, protocol adherence, and timely reporting of adverse events.

2. Scope and Applicability:

- **Trial Coverage:** Clearly outline the scope of the QA Plan, specifying the phases and aspects of the trial it covers, including study design, participant recruitment, data collection, and analysis.

- **Applicability:** Detail which departments, teams, and sites the QA Plan applies to, ensuring comprehensive coverage across the trial.

3. Risk Management:

- **Risk Identification and Assessment:** Incorporate a risk management approach to identify potential risks to the trial's quality and assess their impact and likelihood. Use a risk matrix to prioritize risks and allocate resources effectively.

- **Risk Mitigation Strategies:** Outline strategies and actions to mitigate identified risks, including monitoring plans, training programs, and corrective and preventive actions (CAPA).

4. Standard Operating Procedures (SOPs):

- **Development and Review:** Describe the process for developing, reviewing, and updating SOPs that support the QA Plan. SOPs should cover critical trial processes, data management, safety monitoring, and regulatory compliance.

- **Accessibility:** Ensure that all relevant personnel have easy access to current versions of SOPs and are trained in their application.

5. Training and Competency:

- **Training Programs:** Detail the training programs in place for trial personnel, covering GCP principles, trial-specific procedures, data management systems, and ethical conduct. Include new employee training as well as ongoing education.

- **Competency Assessment:** Outline procedures for assessing the competency of trial staff and investigators, including certifications, qualifications, and performance evaluations.

6. Monitoring and Auditing:

- **Monitoring Plans:** Specify the plans for ongoing monitoring of trial conduct and data quality, including the frequency of monitoring visits, remote monitoring activities, and the use of electronic data capture (EDC) systems for real-time oversight.

- **Independent Audits:** Plan for regular independent audits to assess compliance with the QA Plan, GCP, and regulatory requirements. Include the scope, frequency, and responsibilities for conducting audits.

7. Documentation and Record-keeping:

- **Document Control:** Implement document control procedures to ensure that all trial documentation is accurate, complete, and secure. This includes maintaining an audit trail for document revisions and ensuring compliance with data protection laws.

- **Record Retention:** Define the procedures for the retention, retrieval, and destruction of trial records, in accordance with regulatory requirements and sponsor policies.

8. Communication and Reporting:

- **Communication Channels:** Establish clear channels for communication within the trial team and with external stakeholders (regulatory bodies, ethics committees, sponsors) regarding quality issues, audit findings, and CAPA implementations.

- **Reporting Mechanisms:** Detail the mechanisms for reporting quality issues, non-compliance events, and the outcomes of quality improvement initiatives.

9. Continuous Improvement:

- **Quality Reviews:** Schedule periodic quality reviews to assess the effectiveness of the QA Plan and identify areas for improvement. Use feedback from audits, monitoring visits, and stakeholder input to refine the plan.

- **Adaptation and Updates:** Describe the process for updating the QA Plan in response to changes in regulatory requirements, trial procedures, or identified quality issues.

Developing a comprehensive QA Plan requires careful consideration of the trial's specific needs and challenges, as well as a commitment to maintaining the highest standards of quality and compliance throughout the trial lifecycle.

9.3 Conducting Quality Audits

Quality audits are a critical component of the quality assurance process in clinical trials. They provide an independent evaluation of the conduct of the trial and the compliance with Good Clinical Practice (GCP), regulatory requirements, and the study protocol. Quality audits help identify areas for improvement, ensure participant safety, and maintain data integrity. Here's a guide on conducting quality audits in clinical trials:

1. Planning the Audit:

- **Define the Scope:** Clearly define the scope of the audit, including the specific processes, departments, or aspects of the trial to be evaluated. This could range from trial site operations, data management practices, to the functioning of the trial's monitoring systems.

- **Selecting the Audit Team:** Choose an audit team with the necessary expertise and independence from the trial operations. This team could include internal auditors or external experts.

- **Scheduling:** Plan the audit at a time that minimizes disruption to trial activities, ensuring key personnel are available for interviews and discussions.

2. Preparing for the Audit:

- **Review of Documentation:** Before the audit, review essential trial documents, including the protocol, Investigator's Brochure, consent forms, previous audit reports, and regulatory correspondence.

- **Communication:** Inform the trial site or department being audited about the upcoming audit, including its scope, objectives, and schedule, to ensure cooperation and preparedness.

3. Conducting the Audit:

- **Opening Meeting:** Start with an opening meeting to discuss the audit process, confirm the agenda, and set expectations with the trial team.

- **Document Review and Interviews:** Conduct thorough reviews of trial documents, records, and data. Interview trial staff and investigators to assess their understanding of the trial protocol, GCP requirements, and their specific responsibilities.

- **Observation:** Where applicable, observe trial-related activities to assess adherence to the protocol and SOPs.

- **Note-taking:** Document findings, observations, and any areas of concern or non-compliance during the audit for later analysis.

4. Reporting Audit Findings:

- **Draft Report:** Prepare a draft audit report summarizing the findings, including instances of non-compliance, areas of risk, and good practices observed.

- **Feedback Session:** Present the draft findings to the audited team for feedback, clarification, and discussion. This session can help ensure accuracy and provide immediate awareness of any issues identified.

- **Final Report:** Finalize the audit report, incorporating feedback from the discussion. The report should detail the audit findings, recommendations for corrective and preventive actions (CAPA), and timelines for implementation.

5. Follow-up and Closure:

- **CAPA Implementation:** Monitor the implementation of CAPA plans to address the audit findings, ensuring actions are taken within agreed timelines.

- **Verification:** Conduct follow-up activities, as necessary, to verify that corrective actions have been effectively implemented and that compliance has been achieved.

- **Audit Closure:** Officially close the audit once all corrective actions have been verified and all issues have been satisfactorily resolved.

6. Continuous Improvement:

- **Learning and Improvement:** Use the insights gained from the audit to foster continuous improvement in trial processes and quality management systems. Share lessons learned with the wider organization or trial network to prevent similar issues in future trials.

Conducting quality audits is an essential practice for maintaining the highest standards of clinical trial conduct. It requires careful planning, execution, and follow-up to ensure that trials are conducted in compliance with ethical and regulatory standards, thereby protecting participant safety and ensuring the reliability of trial results.

9.4 Exercise: 10 MCQs with Answers at the End

Multiple Choice Questions:

1. What is the primary purpose of conducting quality audits in clinical trials?

   - A) To assign blame for any errors

   - B) To increase paperwork for the trial team

   - C) To identify areas for improvement and ensure compliance with regulations

   - D) To limit the scope of the trial

2. What should be clearly defined before conducting an audit?

   - A) The favorite colors of the audit team

   - B) The scope of the audit

   - C) The brand of coffee used at the site

   - D) The names of the participants

3. Who should conduct the quality audit?

   - A) The most junior staff member

   - B) An audit team with necessary expertise and independence

   - C) All trial participants

- D) External marketing consultants

4. What is an essential step in preparing for an audit?

   - A) Ignoring previous audit reports

   - B) Planning a surprise audit date

   - C) Review of essential trial documents

   - D) Ensuring only positive findings are reported

5. During an audit, what activity is NOT typically performed?

   - A) Reviewing documents and records

   - B) Conducting interviews with trial staff

   - C) Observing trial-related activities

   - D) Rearranging the office furniture

6. How should audit findings be initially reported?

   - A) Through anonymous letters

   - B) In a draft audit report for feedback

   - C) On social media

   - D) Only verbally in informal settings

7. What is the final step in the audit process?

   - A) Destroying all trial documents

   - B) Hosting a party for the audit team

   - C) Finalizing the audit report with recommendations for CAPA

   - D) Forgetting about the audit findings

8. Follow-up and closure of the audit involve:

   - A) Ignoring the CAPA implementation

   - B) Monitoring the implementation of CAPA plans

   - C) Eliminating all documentation related to the audit

   - D) Never communicating the audit results

9. Quality audits foster continuous improvement by:

   - A) Discouraging feedback and discussions

   - B) Using insights gained to enhance trial processes

   - C) Keeping findings confidential from the trial team

   - D) Focusing solely on past mistakes without planning for improvements

10. The independence of the audit team is crucial because it:

   - A) Ensures the audit process disrupts trial activities

   - B) Guarantees findings will be biased

   - C) Helps ensure objectivity and unbiased reporting of findings

- D) Allows the team to skip detailed reviews

Answers:

1. C) To identify areas for improvement and ensure compliance with regulations

2. B) The scope of the audit

3. B) An audit team with necessary expertise and independence

4. C) Review of essential trial documents

5. D) Rearranging the office furniture

6. B) In a draft audit report for feedback

7. C) Finalizing the audit report with recommendations for CAPA

8. B) Monitoring the implementation of CAPA plans

9. B) Using insights gained to enhance trial processes

10. C) Helps ensure objectivity and unbiased reporting of findings

Chapter 10: Technology in Clinical Trials

10.1 Leveraging Electronic Data Capture Systems

Electronic Data Capture (EDC) systems have revolutionized the way data is collected, managed, and analyzed in clinical trials. These digital platforms offer a range of functionalities that streamline trial processes, enhance data quality, and improve efficiency. Here's a look at how leveraging EDC systems can significantly benefit clinical trials:

1. Real-time Data Entry and Access:

- **Immediate Data Input:** EDC systems allow for the real-time entry of clinical trial data directly at the point of care or through remote monitoring, reducing delays associated with paper-based data collection.

- **Accessible Data:** Authorized trial personnel can access up-to-date trial data from anywhere, facilitating timely decision-making and enhancing collaboration among researchers and sponsors.

2. Improved Data Quality and Integrity:

- **Error Reduction:** EDC systems often include built-in validation rules that check for data entry errors, missing values, and inconsistencies in real-time, prompting immediate correction and significantly reducing the likelihood of errors.

- **Audit Trails:** These systems automatically generate comprehensive audit trails that record every action taken on the data, including who accessed or modified the data, when, and why, thereby enhancing data integrity and facilitating compliance with regulatory standards.

3. Enhanced Compliance with Regulatory Standards:

- **Good Clinical Practice (GCP) Compliance:** EDC systems are designed to meet GCP guidelines and regulatory requirements, ensuring that the trial is conducted in compliance with ethical and legal standards.

- **Security Measures:** Robust data encryption and secure user authentication protocols protect sensitive trial data against unauthorized access and breaches, aligning with data protection regulations.

4. Streamlined Data Management Processes:

- **Centralized Data Repository:** EDC systems provide a centralized platform for storing and managing all trial data, eliminating the redundancy and fragmentation associated with paper records and disparate databases.

- **Efficient Data Queries and Resolutions:** The system can automatically flag data queries based on predefined criteria, facilitating efficient communication between data managers and site personnel to quickly resolve discrepancies.

5. Facilitation of Remote and Decentralized Trials:

- **Remote Data Collection:** EDC systems are integral to the successful execution of remote and decentralized trials, enabling electronic consent, remote patient monitoring, and virtual site visits.

- **Participant Engagement:** Through patient portals integrated into EDC systems, participants can access their own data, receive reminders for medication adherence or upcoming visits, and stay engaged with the trial process.

6. Cost Reduction and Efficiency:

- **Operational Efficiencies:** By automating data collection, management, and reporting processes, EDC systems can significantly reduce the time and labor costs associated with manual data handling and paper-based systems.

- **Scalability:** The digital nature of EDC systems allows for easy scaling of trial operations, accommodating everything from small pilot studies to large, multi-site international trials without substantial increases in cost.

7. Data Analysis and Reporting:

- **Advanced Analytics:** EDC systems often include or integrate with advanced analytics tools that allow for real-time data analysis, enabling faster identification of trends, safety signals, and efficacy markers.

- **Streamlined Reporting:** Automated report generation capabilities facilitate the timely submission of trial data to regulatory authorities, sponsors, and other stakeholders.

Leveraging EDC systems in clinical trials offers profound benefits in terms of efficiency, data quality, compliance, and participant engagement. As technology continues to evolve, the capabilities and advantages of EDC systems are expected to expand, further transforming the landscape of clinical research.

10.2 The Role of Wearables and Mobile Health Devices

Wearable technology and mobile health (mHealth) devices are playing an increasingly significant role in clinical trials, revolutionizing data collection, patient monitoring, and participant engagement. These technologies facilitate the collection of real-time, high-quality data across a broad range of physiological parameters, offering deeper insights into treatment efficacy, safety, and patient health outcomes. Here's an overview of the impact of wearables and mHealth devices in clinical research:

1. Continuous and Remote Data Collection:

- **Real-time Monitoring:** Wearables and mHealth devices enable continuous monitoring of participants in real-time, allowing for the collection of a wide array of health data, including heart rate, physical activity, sleep patterns, and more, outside the clinical setting.

- **Remote Data Collection:** These devices facilitate remote data collection, making it easier to conduct decentralized trials and gather data from participants in their natural living environments, enhancing the convenience for participants and broadening the scope of potential trial enrollees.

2. Improved Data Quality and Quantity:

- **Objective Data:** Wearables and mHealth devices collect objective, quantifiable data that can reduce reliance on subjective patient-reported outcomes, potentially increasing the accuracy and reliability of trial data.

- **Granular Data:** The ability to collect data at high frequencies over extended periods provides a more detailed and comprehensive view of patient health and treatment effects, enhancing the depth and quality of trial data.

3. Enhancing Participant Engagement and Compliance:

- **Participant Engagement:** The use of wearables and mHealth devices can increase participant engagement by actively involving them in the trial process and providing feedback on their health metrics.

- **Improved Compliance:** Features like reminders for medication intake, scheduled activities, or follow-up visits can improve protocol compliance and retention rates by keeping participants informed and engaged.

4. Personalized and Adaptive Trials:

- **Personalized Interventions:** The rich dataset obtained from wearables and mHealth devices allows for the analysis of individual responses to treatments, paving the way for personalized medicine approaches in clinical trials.

- **Adaptive Trial Designs:** Real-time data collection supports adaptive trial designs, where interventions can be modified based on interim data analyses, optimizing trial outcomes and resource utilization.

5. Safety Monitoring:

- **Early Detection of Adverse Events:** Continuous monitoring enables the early detection of potential adverse events or changes in participant health, allowing for prompt intervention and enhancing participant safety.

- **Passive Safety Monitoring:** The passive nature of data collection through wearables and mHealth devices reduces the burden on participants while ensuring continuous safety monitoring.

6. Challenges and Considerations:

- **Data Privacy and Security:** The collection and transmission of health data through wearables and mHealth devices raise significant concerns about data privacy and security. Ensuring compliance with data protection regulations is paramount.

- **Device Validation and Standardization:** Ensuring the accuracy, reliability, and validity of the data collected by wearables and mHealth devices is crucial. Standardization of device specifications and validation against gold-standard measures are necessary to ensure data integrity.

- **Participant Access and Equity:** Consideration must be given to participants' access to the necessary technology and the potential for disparities in technology literacy, which could impact trial participation and equity.

The integration of wearables and mHealth devices into clinical trials offers promising opportunities to enhance data collection, participant engagement, and the overall trial experience. However, addressing the associated challenges and ethical considerations is essential to fully leverage the potential of these technologies in clinical research.

10.3 Implementing Telemedicine and Remote Monitoring

Telemedicine and remote monitoring technologies have emerged as powerful tools in the execution of clinical trials, particularly in enhancing participant access, improving data collection, and ensuring continuous patient care. These technologies allow trial procedures to be conducted remotely, reducing the need for in-person visits and enabling trials to continue in situations where traditional site visits are challenging. Here's how to effectively implement telemedicine and remote monitoring in clinical trials:

1. Integration into Trial Design:

- **Feasibility Assessment:** Evaluate the feasibility of integrating telemedicine and remote monitoring into the trial design, considering factors such as the study population, intervention type, and data collection requirements.

- **Protocol Modification:** Modify the trial protocol to incorporate telemedicine visits and remote monitoring procedures, clearly defining the technologies to be used, the processes for remote data collection, and the criteria for remote vs. in-person visits.

2. Technology Selection and Validation:

- **Select Appropriate Technologies:** Choose telemedicine platforms and remote monitoring devices that meet the trial's specific needs, ensuring they are user-friendly, reliable, and secure.

- **Validation:** Validate the chosen technologies to ensure they provide accurate and reliable data that are equivalent to those collected through traditional methods.

3. Regulatory Compliance and Ethical Considerations:

- **Privacy and Security:** Ensure telemedicine and remote monitoring solutions comply with data privacy and security regulations, such as GDPR in Europe and HIPAA in the United States, to protect participant information.

- **Informed Consent:** Adapt the informed consent process to clearly communicate the use of telemedicine and remote monitoring, including how data will be collected, stored, and used.

4. Training for Trial Staff and Participants:

- **Staff Training:** Provide comprehensive training for trial staff on the use of telemedicine and remote monitoring technologies, including troubleshooting common issues and maintaining data integrity.

- **Participant Training:** Offer training and support for participants to ensure they are comfortable using the technologies and understand how to report data accurately.

5. Infrastructure and Support:

- **Technical Support:** Establish a robust technical support system to assist trial staff and participants with any technology-related issues, ensuring minimal disruption to trial procedures.

- **Internet Access:** Consider the internet access requirements for remote monitoring and telemedicine interventions, providing support or alternatives for participants with limited access.

6. Monitoring and Quality Assurance:

- **Continuous Monitoring:** Implement continuous monitoring of telemedicine and remote monitoring activities to ensure data quality and protocol adherence.

- **Quality Assurance Checks:** Conduct regular quality assurance checks on the data collected remotely, comparing them with traditional data collection methods when possible to ensure consistency and accuracy.

7. Adapting to Challenges:

- **Flexibility:** Be prepared to adapt telemedicine and remote monitoring procedures in response to participant feedback, technical issues, or changes in the trial's needs.

- **Equity and Access:** Address potential disparities in access to technology and internet connectivity among participants, ensuring that telemedicine and remote monitoring do not introduce biases into the trial.

Implementing telemedicine and remote monitoring in clinical trials requires careful planning, attention to regulatory and ethical considerations, and a commitment to maintaining data quality and participant safety. When effectively integrated, these technologies can significantly enhance the flexibility, efficiency, and reach of clinical trials, opening up new possibilities for research and patient care.

10.4 Exercise: 10 MCQs with Answers at the End

Multiple Choice Questions:

1. What is a key benefit of integrating telemedicine into clinical trials?

  - A) Increasing the need for in-person visits

- B) Enhancing participant access and reducing the need for in-person visits

- C) Complicating the trial protocol

- D) Limiting participant engagement

2. Before implementing telemedicine, what must be evaluated in a clinical trial?

- A) The color scheme of the telemedicine platform

- B) Feasibility and compatibility with the trial design

- C) The preference for traditional methods by all participants

- D) The trial's budget surplus

3. When selecting technologies for remote monitoring, what is crucial?

- A) Choosing the most expensive option

- B) User-friendliness and reliability

- C) The color and design of the devices

- D) Selecting devices without digital displays

4. To protect participant information in telemedicine and remote monitoring, compliance with which regulations is necessary?

   - A) Fashion and design regulations

   - B) Data privacy and security regulations, such as GDPR and HIPAA

   - C) Agricultural standards

   - D) Local culinary guidelines

5. What type of training is essential for the success of telemedicine in clinical trials?

   - A) Only trial staff need training on technology use

   - B) Only participants need training on technology use

   - C) Training for both trial staff and participants on technology use

   - D) No training is necessary

6. What infrastructure consideration is important for telemedicine interventions?

   - A) Ensuring all participants have a landline phone

   - B) Providing high-speed internet access where necessary

   - C) Making sure all participants live in urban areas

   - D) Guaranteeing that all communication happens via fax

7. Continuous monitoring in telemedicine and remote monitoring is implemented to ensure what?

 - A) Data quality and protocol adherence

 - B) The social media popularity of the trial

 - C) That all communications are recorded for entertainment

 - D) Increasing the complexity of data analysis

8. Which strategy helps address technology and connectivity disparities among participants in telemedicine-based trials?

 - A) Ignoring disparities as irrelevant

 - B) Ensuring access and support for all participants

 - C) Only selecting participants with high-speed internet

 - D) Using only non-digital communication methods

9. What aspect of telemedicine and remote monitoring must be adapted based on participant feedback and technical issues?

 - A) The trial's primary endpoint

 - B) The color theme of the telemedicine platform

 - C) The procedural aspects and technologies used

 - D) The geographical location of the trial

10. Ensuring compliance with what is paramount when using telemedicine and remote monitoring technologies?

   - A) Only internal trial policies, ignoring external regulations

   - B) Data privacy and security regulations

   - C) Personal preferences of the trial staff

   - D) The most recent fashion trends

Answers:

1. B) Enhancing participant access and reducing the need for in-person visits

2. B) Feasibility and compatibility with the trial design

3. B) User-friendliness and reliability

4. B) Data privacy and security regulations, such as GDPR and HIPAA

5. C) Training for both trial staff and participants on technology use

6. B) Providing high-speed internet access where necessary

7. A) Data quality and protocol adherence

8. B) Ensuring access and support for all participants

9. C) The procedural aspects and technologies used

10. B) Data privacy and security regulations

Chapter 11: Managing Clinical Trial Teams

11.1 Building and Leading Effective Teams

Effective team management is crucial in clinical trials, as it directly impacts the study's success, efficiency, and adherence to ethical and regulatory standards. Building and leading a cohesive, motivated, and skilled clinical trial team requires understanding diverse roles, fostering communication, and creating a supportive work environment. Here are key strategies for building and leading effective clinical trial teams:

1. Define Clear Roles and Responsibilities:

- **Role Clarity:** Clearly define the roles and responsibilities of each team member, ensuring that their duties align with their skills and experience. This clarity helps in minimizing overlaps and gaps in responsibilities, leading to more efficient team functioning.

- **Expectation Setting:** Set clear expectations for performance, communication, and adherence to protocols and regulations, establishing a standard for accountability.

2. Foster a Collaborative Team Culture:

- **Open Communication:** Encourage open and honest communication within the team. Regular meetings, updates, and feedback sessions can foster a sense of collaboration and transparency.

- **Respect and Inclusion:** Promote a culture of respect, inclusivity, and diversity, recognizing and valuing the unique contributions of each team member. This environment can boost morale and encourage innovation.

3. Invest in Team Development:

- **Training and Education:** Provide ongoing training and professional development opportunities for team members to enhance their skills, knowledge, and competency in clinical trial management.

- **Career Pathways:** Offer clear career development pathways and growth opportunities within the organization to motivate and retain talented team members.

4. Effective Leadership:

- **Lead by Example:** Demonstrate commitment, integrity, and professionalism. Leaders who exemplify the qualities they expect from their team members can inspire and motivate their teams more effectively.

- **Adaptive Leadership:** Be prepared to adapt leadership styles based on the team's needs, project phase, and individual team members' preferences to effectively manage and guide the team through challenges.

5. Promote Team Well-being and Work-Life Balance:

- **Supportive Environment:** Create a supportive work environment that recognizes the importance of mental health and work-life balance. Acknowledging the pressures of clinical trial work and offering support can reduce burnout and improve team satisfaction.

- **Flexibility:** Where possible, offer flexible working arrangements to accommodate the personal needs of team members, enhancing their engagement and loyalty.

6. Encourage Problem-Solving and Innovation:

- **Empowerment:** Empower team members to take initiative and make decisions within their areas of responsibility. Encouraging autonomy can lead to innovative solutions to trial challenges.

- **Collaborative Problem-Solving:** Promote a problem-solving approach that encourages team members to collaborate on identifying issues, brainstorming solutions, and implementing improvements.

7. Recognize and Reward Contributions:

- **Acknowledgment:** Regularly acknowledge and celebrate the achievements and contributions of team members, both individually and as a group. Recognition can significantly boost morale and motivation.

- **Reward Systems:** Implement reward systems that align with team and individual performance goals, further incentivizing high performance and dedication.

Building and leading effective clinical trial teams is a dynamic and ongoing process that requires attention to individual and collective needs, clear communication, and strong leadership. By implementing these strategies, team leaders can foster a productive, engaged, and collaborative team capable of navigating the complexities of clinical trial management successfully.

11.2 Communication Strategies for Team Management

Effective communication is the backbone of successful team management, especially in the intricate and high-stakes environment of clinical trials. Clear, consistent, and open communication fosters teamwork, enhances problem-solving, and ensures alignment with the trial's goals and protocols. Here are essential communication strategies for managing clinical trial teams:

1. Establish Clear Communication Channels:

- **Defined Channels:** Specify formal and informal channels for team communication, such as meetings, emails, instant messaging platforms, and internal collaboration tools. Clear channels help prevent information silos and ensure that important information reaches all relevant team members.

- **Accessibility:** Ensure that communication channels are accessible to all team members, considering remote or part-time staff, to foster inclusivity.

2. Regular Meetings and Updates:

- **Scheduled Meetings:** Hold regular team meetings to discuss trial progress, address issues, and share updates. This could include daily stand-ups, weekly team meetings, and monthly all-hands meetings.

- **Agendas and Minutes:** Prepare agendas in advance and distribute minutes after meetings to document discussions and action items, ensuring that team members are aligned and accountable.

3. Transparent and Open Communication:

- **Encourage Openness:** Cultivate an environment where team members feel comfortable sharing ideas, concerns, and feedback. An open-door policy by leaders can encourage this.

- **Transparency:** Be transparent about trial progress, challenges, and changes in protocols or objectives. Transparency builds trust and ensures that the team can adapt to new information.

4. Tailored Communication:

- **Understand Your Audience:** Tailor communication styles and methods to the preferences and needs of different team members. Consider cultural differences, language barriers, and personal preferences to enhance understanding and engagement.

- **Feedback Mechanisms:** Implement mechanisms for team members to provide feedback on communication effectiveness and suggest improvements.

5. Effective Use of Technology:

- **Collaboration Tools:** Utilize technology and collaboration tools to facilitate communication, especially for remote or geographically dispersed teams. Tools like project management software, video conferencing, and secure document sharing can enhance collaboration and efficiency.

- **Training on Tools:** Provide training on how to use communication and collaboration technologies to ensure all team members can participate fully.

6. Conflict Resolution:

- **Proactive Conflict Management:** Address conflicts and misunderstandings promptly through open dialogue and mediation. Establishing clear procedures for conflict resolution can help manage disagreements constructively.

- **Positive Reinforcement:** Focus on positive reinforcement and solutions rather than blame, fostering a supportive team atmosphere.

7. Celebrating Successes:

- **Recognition:** Regularly recognize and celebrate team successes and milestones, both big and small. Acknowledging achievements can boost morale and reinforce the value of team efforts.

- **Team Building:** Organize team-building activities that allow team members to connect on a personal level, strengthening relationships and improving team dynamics.

Implementing these communication strategies can significantly enhance team cohesion, productivity, and satisfaction. Effective communication not only supports the logistical aspects of conducting a clinical trial but also builds a supportive and collaborative team culture that can navigate the complexities and challenges of clinical research.

11.3 Conflict Resolution and Problem Solving

Conflicts and challenges are inevitable in the complex and high-pressure environment of clinical trials. Effective conflict resolution and problem-solving are essential skills for team leaders to maintain team cohesion, ensure project progress, and uphold a positive work environment. Here's a guide to navigating conflict resolution and problem-solving in clinical trial teams:

1. Early Identification and Acknowledgment:

- **Proactive Observation:** Be vigilant for signs of conflict or emerging problems within the team, such as communication breakdowns, decreased productivity, or expressions of frustration.

- **Acknowledgment:** Acknowledge the issue early and openly, validating the concerns of those involved without assigning blame, to prevent escalation and foster an environment where challenges are addressed constructively.

2. Open Communication and Active Listening:

- **Encourage Open Dialogue:** Create a safe and private space for open dialogue, encouraging all parties involved to share their perspectives and feelings on the matter.

- **Active Listening:** Practice active listening, where you attentively listen to understand, not just to respond. This helps in fully understanding the root causes of the conflict or problem.

3. Analyze the Issue:

- **Objective Assessment:** Together with the team, objectively assess the issue, separating personal feelings from professional concerns. Focus on identifying the underlying causes of the conflict or problem.

- **Impact Evaluation:** Consider the impact of the issue on the team's dynamics, the trial's progress, and individual well-being to gauge the urgency and scale of the required resolution.

4. Collaborative Problem-Solving:

- **Inclusive Approach:** Engage all relevant team members in brainstorming potential solutions. A collaborative approach ensures that solutions are comprehensive and consider different perspectives.

- **Solution Selection:** Together, evaluate the proposed solutions based on feasibility, potential impact, and alignment with trial goals. Agree on a plan of action that addresses the root cause and is acceptable to all parties involved.

5. Implement and Monitor the Resolution:

- **Action Plan:** Develop a clear action plan with defined roles, responsibilities, and timelines for implementing the agreed-upon solution.

- **Monitoring:** Monitor the implementation of the solution and its effectiveness in resolving the issue. Be open to adjusting the plan as needed based on feedback and observed outcomes.

6. Learning and Improvement:

- **Reflection:** After the resolution, reflect on the conflict or problem-solving process to identify learning opportunities. Discuss what worked well, what didn't, and why.

- **Continuous Improvement:** Use the insights gained to improve team communication, workflows, and conflict resolution strategies. Consider implementing preventive measures to avoid similar issues in the future.

7. Maintain Professionalism and Respect:

- **Respectful Interactions:** Throughout the conflict resolution and problem-solving process, maintain professionalism, respect, and confidentiality. This helps preserve relationships and trust among team members.

- **Supportive Environment:** Foster a supportive team environment that values constructive feedback, mutual respect, and continuous learning.

Effective conflict resolution and problem-solving require patience, empathy, and strong leadership. By addressing issues constructively and collaboratively, team leaders can navigate challenges, minimize their impact on the clinical trial, and strengthen the team's resilience and cohesion.

11.4 Exercise: 10 MCQs with Answers at the End

Multiple Choice Questions:

1. What is the first step in effective conflict resolution in clinical trial teams?

   - A) Assigning blame to involved parties

   - B) Ignoring the conflict hoping it resolves itself

   - C) Early identification and acknowledgment of the issue

   - D) Immediately informing external authorities

2. Which skill is crucial for understanding the root causes of a conflict?

- A) Negotiation

- B) Active listening

- C) Persuasion

- D) Public speaking

3. When analyzing an issue, what is important to separate from professional concerns?

- A) Personal feelings

- B) Data analysis

- C) Budget considerations

- D) Trial outcomes

4. In collaborative problem-solving, how should solutions be evaluated?

- A) Based on who proposed them

- B) By their complexity

- C) Based on feasibility and impact

- D) According to the highest cost

5. What is essential after implementing a resolution?

- A) Monitoring its effectiveness

- B) Taking a vacation

- C) Avoiding further communication on the matter

- D) Celebrating regardless of the outcome

6. What practice helps in learning from the conflict resolution process?

- A) Reflection on the process

- B) Forgetting about the issue as soon as it's resolved

- C) Never discussing the conflict again

- D) Only focusing on negative outcomes

7. Which approach is least effective in maintaining team cohesion during conflicts?

- A) Maintaining professionalism and respect

- B) Active listening and open dialogue

- C) Using conflicts as learning opportunities

- D) Ignoring conflicts and avoiding discussions

8. What environment fosters constructive feedback and continuous learning?

- A) A competitive environment

- B) A supportive team environment

- C) An isolated work environment

- D) A high-pressure environment

9. Effective conflict resolution and problem-solving require what kind of leadership?

- A) Passive leadership

- B) Dictatorial leadership

- C) Empathetic and strong leadership

- D) Absent leadership

10. Which of the following is not a benefit of effective conflict resolution?

- A) Strengthened team resilience and cohesion

- B) Increased frequency of conflicts

- C) Minimized impact on the trial

- D) Improved team communication and workflows

Answers:

1. C) Early identification and acknowledgment of the issue

2. B) Active listening

3. A) Personal feelings

4. C) Based on feasibility and impact

5. A) Monitoring its effectiveness

6. A) Reflection on the process

7. D) Ignoring conflicts and avoiding discussions

8. B) A supportive team environment

9. C) Empathetic and strong leadership

10. B) Increased frequency of conflicts

Chapter 12: Stakeholder Engagement and Communication

12.1 Identifying Key Stakeholders

Effective stakeholder engagement is crucial in clinical trials to ensure the trial is conducted efficiently, ethically, and in compliance with regulatory requirements. Identifying key stakeholders early in the trial process allows for better communication, collaboration, and alignment of goals. Here's a guide to identifying key stakeholders in clinical trials:

1. Trial Participants:

- The most important stakeholders, their safety, well-being, and rights are the primary concern of any clinical trial. Engaging participants involves clear communication about the trial's purpose, procedures, risks, and benefits.

2. Regulatory Authorities:

- Bodies like the FDA (U.S.), EMA (Europe), and others globally are responsible for overseeing the conduct of clinical trials to ensure they meet regulatory standards. Early and ongoing communication with these authorities is essential for regulatory compliance.

3. Institutional Review Boards (IRBs)/Ethics Committees:

- These groups review and approve the ethical aspects of the clinical trial, focusing on participant safety and rights. Their approval is necessary to initiate and continue the trial.

4. Trial Sponsors:

- Often pharmaceutical, biotechnology companies, or academic institutions, sponsors fund the trial and have a vested interest in its outcome. They play a key role in trial design, implementation, and analysis.

5. Clinical Trial Investigators and Site Staff:

- Investigators lead the trial at each site, and along with the site staff, play a crucial role in executing the trial protocol, managing participant care, and collecting data.

6. Contract Research Organizations (CROs):

- CROs are often employed by sponsors to manage the day-to-day operations of a trial. They work closely with sites and other stakeholders to ensure the trial meets its objectives efficiently.

7. Patient Advocacy Groups:

- These groups represent the interests of patients and can aid in participant recruitment, provide input on trial design to ensure it meets patient needs, and help disseminate trial results.

8. Healthcare Providers:

- Physicians and healthcare providers not directly involved in the trial may refer patients to participate or provide care to participants. Keeping them informed about the trial can facilitate referrals and ensure continuity of care.

9. Academic and Research Institutions:

- For trials affiliated with academic institutions, these entities may have an interest in the trial's conduct and outcomes for research, educational, and reputational purposes.

10. Third-party Vendors and Technology Providers:

- Vendors providing technology solutions, laboratory services, and other essential services are stakeholders whose performance can directly impact trial outcomes.

11. Local Communities and the General Public:

- Especially for trials with significant public health implications, the broader community and public may have a stake in the trial's conduct and outcomes.

Identifying and understanding the roles, interests, and influence of these stakeholders are crucial steps in planning and executing a successful clinical trial. Effective stakeholder engagement involves tailored communication strategies, collaborative planning, and feedback mechanisms to align the trial's goals with the expectations and needs of all involved parties.

12.2 Effective Communication Strategies

Effective communication with stakeholders is essential for the success of clinical trials. It ensures transparency, fosters trust, facilitates collaboration, and enhances trial outcomes. Here are key strategies for effective communication with clinical trial stakeholders:

1. Develop a Communication Plan:

- **Tailored Messaging:** Create a comprehensive communication plan that outlines key messages tailored to the interests and needs of different stakeholder groups. This plan should include objectives, channels, frequency, and responsible parties for each communication activity.

- **Feedback Mechanisms:** Incorporate mechanisms for stakeholders to provide feedback, ask questions, and express concerns, enabling two-way communication.

2. Utilize Multiple Channels:

- **Diverse Channels:** Employ a variety of communication channels to reach stakeholders effectively. These can include emails, newsletters, websites, social media, virtual meetings, and in-person events.

- **Accessibility:** Ensure that communication channels are accessible to all stakeholders, considering factors like language, technology access, and disabilities.

3. Ensure Clarity and Transparency:

- **Clear and Concise Information:** Communicate in clear, concise, and jargon-free language to ensure that all stakeholders can understand the information provided, regardless of their background in clinical research.

- **Transparency:** Be transparent about trial objectives, processes, risks, benefits, and progress. Transparency builds trust and helps manage stakeholders' expectations.

4. Regular Updates and Reporting:

- **Progress Updates:** Provide regular updates on trial progress, milestones reached, and any challenges or changes to the trial. This keeps stakeholders informed and engaged throughout the trial's lifecycle.

- **Reporting Results:** Share trial results in a timely and responsible manner, acknowledging the contributions of all stakeholders, especially participants.

5. Tailored Communication for Different Stakeholders:

- **Participants:** Focus on informed consent processes, trial procedures, potential risks and benefits, and updates on trial progress and results.

- **Regulatory Authorities and IRBs:** Provide detailed documentation and reports as required, ensuring compliance with regulatory standards and guidelines.

- **Sponsors:** Maintain open lines of communication regarding trial progress, financial aspects, and any issues that may impact trial outcomes.

- **Site Staff and Investigators:** Offer training, protocol updates, and forums for discussion and problem-solving.

- **Patient Advocacy Groups:** Engage in dialogue about patient needs and perspectives, and utilize their networks for participant recruitment and dissemination of results.

6. Training and Support:

- **Communication Skills Training:** Provide training for team members responsible for stakeholder communication to enhance their skills in effective, empathetic, and clear communication.

- **Support Materials:** Develop support materials, such as FAQs, information leaflets, and tutorial videos, to assist stakeholders in understanding the trial and their roles within it.

7. Conflict Resolution:

- **Proactive Approach:** Address conflicts or misunderstandings promptly through open dialogue, seeking to understand all perspectives and working collaboratively towards resolutions.

8. Celebrate and Acknowledge Contributions:

- **Recognition:** Acknowledge and celebrate the contributions of all stakeholders, particularly trial participants and site staff, reinforcing their value to the trial's success.

Effective communication in clinical trials requires planning, adaptability, and a commitment to transparency and inclusivity. By employing these strategies, trial managers can build strong relationships with stakeholders, enhancing cooperation, trust, and ultimately, the success of the trial.

12.3 Managing Expectations and Relationships

Managing expectations and relationships with stakeholders is crucial in clinical trials to ensure smooth operations, foster trust, and maintain a positive and productive working environment. Here's how to effectively manage expectations and relationships in the context of clinical trials:

1. Set Clear Expectations Early:

- **Transparent Communication:** From the onset, communicate clearly about the trial's objectives, processes, timelines, and potential risks and benefits. Setting realistic expectations helps prevent misunderstandings and disappointment.

- **Informed Consent:** For trial participants, the informed consent process is critical for setting expectations regarding their involvement, the procedures they will undergo, potential risks, and their rights.

2. Regular and Open Communication:

- **Continuous Updates:** Provide regular updates to all stakeholders about trial progress, any changes to the trial protocol, and preliminary findings. Keeping stakeholders informed helps manage their expectations and reinforces their trust in the trial management.

- **Feedback Mechanisms:** Establish mechanisms for stakeholders to ask questions, express concerns, and provide feedback. Addressing stakeholder inquiries promptly and effectively is key to maintaining positive relationships.

3. Understand Stakeholder Perspectives:

- **Stakeholder Engagement:** Engage with stakeholders to understand their interests, concerns, and expectations. This can involve one-on-one meetings, focus groups, or surveys.

- **Empathy:** Show empathy towards stakeholders' perspectives and concerns. Acknowledging and addressing these can foster stronger relationships and enhance collaboration.

4. Manage Conflicts Proactively:

- **Conflict Identification:** Be vigilant in identifying potential conflicts or disagreements early. Proactive management can prevent escalation and maintain a collaborative atmosphere.

- **Resolution Strategies:** Employ conflict resolution strategies that focus on open dialogue, understanding differing perspectives, and finding mutually acceptable solutions.

5. Adaptability and Flexibility:

- **Responding to Changes:** Clinical trials can be unpredictable, with changes in regulations, protocols, or unexpected challenges. Be prepared to adapt strategies and communicate these changes effectively to stakeholders.

- **Flexibility in Expectations:** Help stakeholders understand the need for flexibility in expectations due to the dynamic nature of clinical trials.

6. Build and Maintain Trust:

- **Consistency and Reliability:** Be consistent and reliable in your communications and actions. Consistency builds trust over time, which is essential for effective stakeholder relationships.

- **Transparency:** Be transparent about challenges, uncertainties, and mistakes. Transparency in difficult times can strengthen trust and credibility.

7. Recognize and Value Contributions:

- **Acknowledgment:** Regularly acknowledge and express appreciation for the contributions of all stakeholders, particularly trial participants and site staff. Recognition can enhance motivation and commitment to the trial.

- **Celebrating Milestones:** Celebrate key milestones and successes with stakeholders to foster a sense of shared achievement and belonging.

8. Foster a Collaborative Environment:

- **Encourage Collaboration:** Promote a culture of collaboration and teamwork among stakeholders. Collaborative efforts can lead to innovative solutions and a more successful trial outcome.

Managing expectations and relationships in clinical trials requires ongoing effort, sensitivity to stakeholder needs, and a commitment to open and honest communication. By employing these strategies, trial managers can navigate the complexities of clinical trials while fostering strong and productive relationships with all involved parties.

12.4 Exercise: 10 MCQs with Answers at the End

Multiple Choice Questions:

1. What is the foundation of effective stakeholder engagement in clinical trials?

   - A) Ignoring stakeholder feedback

   - B) Effective communication

   - C) Limiting information shared

   - D) Only focusing on regulatory authorities

2. Tailoring communication to different stakeholders is important because:

   - A) It ensures regulatory compliance

- B) Different stakeholders have unique interests and information needs

   - C) It's a requirement of all clinical trials

   - D) Stakeholders prefer generic messages

3. Regular updates and progress reports to stakeholders serve to:

   - A) Fulfill a legal obligation

   - B) Keep stakeholders informed and engaged

   - C) Overwhelm stakeholders with data

   - D) Reduce transparency in trial processes

4. Which strategy is NOT effective for managing expectations in clinical trials?

   - A) Setting unrealistic goals for trial outcomes

   - B) Being transparent about trial processes and potential risks

   - C) Regularly updating stakeholders on trial progress

   - D) Acknowledging stakeholder contributions

5. Conflict resolution in stakeholder communication should prioritize:

   - A) Finding who is to blame

   - B) Immediate solutions without understanding the issue

   - C) Open dialogue and understanding all perspectives

   - D) Ignoring conflicts to avoid tension

6. The role of training in stakeholder communication is to:

   - A) Increase the complexity of information shared

   - B) Enhance skills in effective and empathetic communication

   - C) Decrease the frequency of communication

   - D) Focus solely on legal and regulatory aspects

7. Utilizing multiple communication channels helps to:

   - A) Complicate the communication process

   - B) Ensure messages reach all relevant stakeholders effectively

   - C) Limit stakeholder engagement to digital platforms only

   - D) Increase the trial's budget unnecessarily

8. Feedback mechanisms in communication plans are essential for:

   - A) Gathering stakeholder criticisms only

- B) Facilitating two-way communication and continuous improvement

   - C) Discouraging stakeholder participation in decision-making

   - D) Simplifying message content to a one-size-fits-all approach

9. Celebrating successes and acknowledging contributions in clinical trials is important to:

   - A) Meet regulatory requirements

- B) Motivate and reinforce the value of stakeholders' involvement

   - C) Highlight the superiority of the trial team

   - D) Shift focus away from any trial failures

10. The main goal of managing expectations in clinical trials is to:

   - A) Create hype around the trial results

   - B) Ensure stakeholders have a realistic understanding of trial processes, timelines, and potential outcomes

   - C) Avoid sharing detailed trial information

   - D) Prioritize sponsor expectations over others

Answers:

1. B) Effective communication

2. B) Different stakeholders have unique interests and information needs

3. B) Keep stakeholders informed and engaged

4. A) Setting unrealistic goals for trial outcomes

5. C) Open dialogue and understanding all perspectives

6. B) Enhance skills in effective and empathetic communication

7. B) Ensure messages reach all relevant stakeholders effectively

8. B) Facilitating two-way communication and continuous improvement

9. B) Motivate and reinforce the value of stakeholders' involvement

10. B) Ensure stakeholders have a realistic understanding of trial processes, timelines, and potential outcomes

Chapter 13: Global Clinical Trials

13.1 Challenges and Opportunities in Global Trials

Global clinical trials, which are conducted across multiple countries and regions, offer unique opportunities for expanding patient access, enhancing diversity in research, and accelerating drug development. However, these trials also present a set of challenges that require careful management to ensure success. Here's an overview of the challenges and opportunities in conducting global clinical trials:

Challenges in Global Clinical Trials:

1. **Regulatory Compliance:**

   - Each country has its own regulatory body and guidelines, making compliance a complex task. Ensuring that the trial meets the requirements of local regulations while maintaining consistency across sites is challenging.

2. Cultural and Linguistic Differences:

   - Variations in language, culture, and healthcare practices can impact participant recruitment, informed consent processes, and data collection methods. Tailoring approaches to suit local contexts is essential but resource-intensive.

3. Logistical Coordination:

   - Managing logistics across different time zones, including the shipment of trial materials, coordination of data collection, and monitoring activities, requires robust planning and communication infrastructure.

4. Ethical Considerations:

   - Ethical standards may vary across regions. Ensuring that the trial upholds the highest ethical standards internationally, especially in vulnerable populations, is paramount.

5. Data Management and Integration:

   - Harmonizing data collected from diverse settings and ensuring its quality and integrity pose significant challenges, especially when different electronic data capture (EDC) systems are used.

Opportunities in Global Clinical Trials:

1. Access to Diverse Patient Populations:

- Conducting trials globally allows access to a broader and more diverse patient population, which can enhance the generalizability of trial results and facilitate the study of rare diseases.

2. Accelerated Recruitment:

- Access to large, diverse patient pools across multiple regions can accelerate participant recruitment, reducing the overall timeline of the trial.

3. Operational Efficiencies:

- Global trials offer the opportunity to leverage differences in cost structures across countries, potentially reducing the overall cost of the trial. Furthermore, the ability to conduct trials in regions with differing seasonal disease patterns can ensure continuous data collection.

4. Enhanced Data Richness:

- Global trials can provide valuable insights into the efficacy and safety of interventions across different genetic backgrounds, lifestyles, and healthcare settings, enriching the understanding of the intervention's impact.

5. **Regulatory and Market Advantages:**

- Conducting trials in key markets can facilitate regulatory submissions and market access post-approval. Engaging with global regulatory authorities early in the trial design can streamline the approval process across multiple jurisdictions.

Strategies for Success:

- **Global Collaboration:** Foster strong collaborations between sponsors, CROs, local investigators, and regulatory authorities to navigate the complexities of global trials effectively.

- **Cultural Competence:** Invest in cultural competence training for trial staff to enhance communication and engagement with participants from diverse backgrounds.

- **Robust Infrastructure:** Develop a robust infrastructure for data management, logistics coordination, and communication that can support the complexities of a global trial network.

- **Ethical Commitment:** Maintain a strong commitment to ethical standards, ensuring that all trial activities respect local customs, laws, and participant rights.

Global clinical trials offer significant opportunities to advance medical research and improve patient outcomes worldwide. By carefully managing the associated challenges, researchers can harness the full potential of global trials to bring effective and safe treatments to the market more efficiently.

13.2 Navigating International Regulations

Conducting clinical trials on a global scale involves navigating a complex web of international regulations and guidelines. Each country or region has its own regulatory framework governing clinical trials, making compliance a significant challenge but also a critical aspect of global trial success. Here's a guide to navigating international regulations in global clinical trials:

1. Understand Local Regulatory Landscapes:

- **Comprehensive Research:** Begin with thorough research to understand the regulatory requirements in each country or region where the trial will be conducted. This includes submission processes, required documentation, timelines, and ethical review procedures.

- **Regulatory Authorities:** Identify the relevant regulatory authorities in each location, such as the FDA (United States), EMA (European Union), MHRA (United Kingdom), and PMDA (Japan), and understand their specific requirements and expectations.

2. Harmonization Efforts and Guidelines:

- **ICH Guidelines:** Familiarize yourself with the International Council for Harmonisation of Technical Requirements for

Pharmaceuticals for Human Use (ICH) guidelines, particularly ICH E6 (R2) Good Clinical Practice, which aim to bring consistency to the regulatory requirements of major markets.

- **Global Harmonization Task Force (GHTF):** For medical devices, refer to the guidelines from the GHTF, which seeks to standardize regulatory practices around the world.

3. Ethical Considerations:

- **Declaration of Helsinki:** Ensure that the trial design and conduct adhere to the ethical principles outlined in the Declaration of Helsinki, which is widely recognized internationally.

- **Local Ethics Committees:** Beyond regulatory approvals, obtain clearance from local ethics committees or institutional review boards (IRBs), which may have additional requirements or concerns specific to the local context.

4. Engagement with Regulatory Authorities:

- **Early Communication:** Engage with regulatory authorities early in the trial planning process. Early and open communication can help clarify requirements, identify potential issues, and facilitate smoother submissions.

- **Consultations and Pre-submission Meetings:** Utilize any opportunities for consultations or pre-submission meetings with regulatory bodies to gain insights into their expectations and receive guidance on submission strategies.

5. Adaptation to Local Requirements:

- **Trial Documentation:** Prepare trial documentation, including protocols, informed consent forms, and investigator brochures, to meet the specific requirements of each regulatory authority. This may involve translations and adaptations to reflect local legal and cultural considerations.

- **Data Protection Laws:** Comply with local data protection laws and regulations, such as GDPR in Europe, which govern the collection, use, and storage of participant data.

6. Monitoring and Compliance:

- **Regulatory Monitoring:** Establish a process for ongoing monitoring of regulatory changes in each country or region throughout the trial duration, as regulations and guidelines can evolve.

- **Audit Preparedness:** Maintain audit-ready documentation and processes to demonstrate compliance with both international and local regulations during inspections or audits by regulatory authorities.

7. Leveraging Expertise:

- **Local Partners and CROs:** Consider partnering with local CROs or experts who have in-depth knowledge of the regulatory environment and established relationships with local regulatory authorities to navigate the approval process more efficiently.

Navigating international regulations in global clinical trials requires a proactive, informed approach and a commitment to maintaining high ethical and quality standards. By understanding and respecting the regulatory landscape of each location, trial sponsors can facilitate regulatory approvals, ensuring the global trial's success and integrity.

13.3 Cultural Considerations and Ethical Standards

Global clinical trials necessitate a nuanced understanding of cultural considerations and adherence to ethical standards across diverse geographical locations. These elements are critical not only for regulatory compliance but also for ensuring the respect, safety, and engagement of trial participants worldwide. Here's how to navigate these aspects in global clinical trials:

1. Cultural Sensitivity in Clinical Trials:

- **Understanding Cultural Norms:** Research and understand the cultural norms, beliefs, and practices of the participant populations in each trial location. This understanding should inform trial design, communication strategies, informed consent processes, and participant interactions.

- **Language and Communication:** Ensure that all trial-related documents and communications are accurately translated into the local languages and that they consider literacy levels and cultural nuances. Use of professional translators and cultural consultants is recommended.

- **Respecting Local Customs:** Adapt trial procedures to respect local customs and practices, where possible, to facilitate participant comfort and engagement. This may include considerations around gender norms, religious practices, and community hierarchies.

2. Ethical Standards Across Regions:

- **Universal Ethical Principles:** Adhere to universally recognized ethical principles, such as those outlined in the Declaration of Helsinki, including respect for persons, beneficence, and justice.

- **Local Ethics Review:** Obtain approval from local ethics committees or institutional review boards (IRBs), ensuring that the trial meets both international and local ethical standards. Local ethics bodies may provide valuable insights into cultural and ethical considerations specific to their communities.

3. Informed Consent Process:

- **Culturally Appropriate Consent:** Tailor the informed consent process to align with cultural norms and practices, ensuring that participants fully understand the trial, their rights, and the potential risks and benefits. This may involve verbal consent processes or community consent in cultures where written consent is not the norm.

- **Ongoing Consent:** Recognize informed consent as an ongoing process, requiring continuous communication and re-affirmation, particularly in cultures where initial consent may not imply continued agreement over time.

4. Community Engagement:

- **Building Relationships with Communities:** Engage with local communities and stakeholders early in the trial planning process to build trust, understand community concerns, and foster collaboration.

- **Community Advisory Boards:** Consider establishing community advisory boards to provide ongoing input on trial conduct, helping to ensure that the trial is conducted in a manner that is respectful and responsive to local needs and values.

5. Addressing Health Inequities:

- **Equitable Access:** Strive for equitable access to trial participation, ensuring that underserved or marginalized populations have opportunities to participate and benefit from the research.

- **Benefit Sharing:** Plan for the sharing of trial benefits with participant communities, such as access to successful interventions, healthcare improvements, or capacity building, to contribute to long-term health equity.

6. Training for Trial Teams:

- **Cultural Competence Training:** Provide cultural competence training for trial teams, equipping them with the skills to interact sensitively and effectively with participants from diverse cultural backgrounds.

- **Ethical Training:** Ensure that all team members are trained in ethical research conduct, with a strong emphasis on respecting participant rights, ensuring informed consent, and protecting participant welfare.

Navigating cultural considerations and ethical standards in global clinical trials is essential for conducting respectful, equitable, and successful research. By prioritizing cultural sensitivity and ethical integrity, researchers can enhance participant engagement, ensure regulatory compliance, and ultimately contribute to the global advancement of medical knowledge and healthcare.

13.4 Exercise: 10 MCQs with Answers at the End

Multiple Choice Questions:

1. Cultural considerations in global clinical trials are important for:

- A) Increasing trial costs.

- B) Ensuring respect for local norms and participant engagement.

- C) Simplifying trial protocols.

- D) Limiting trial locations to culturally homogenous areas.

2. The Declaration of Helsinki is a set of ethical guidelines that emphasizes:

- A) The financial benefits of clinical trials.

- B) The use of placebo in all trials.

- C) Respect for persons, beneficence, and justice.

- D) The priority of sponsor interests.

3. Tailoring the informed consent process in global clinical trials involves:

- A) Providing information exclusively in the trial team's preferred language.

- B) Ignoring local languages and literacy levels.

- C) Adjusting to cultural norms and ensuring comprehension.

- D) Using complex medical jargon to impress participants.

4. Community engagement in the context of global trials often includes:

   - A) Avoiding any contact with the local community.

   - B) Building trust and fostering collaboration with local communities.

   - C) Solely focusing on recruitment without community feedback.

   - D) Making unilateral decisions without community input.

5. Addressing health inequities in global clinical trials is crucial for:

   - A) Ensuring the wealthiest participants benefit the most.

   - B) Providing equitable access and benefit sharing with participant communities.

   - C) Focusing solely on urban populations.

   - D) Excluding underserved and marginalized populations.

6. The ongoing consent process is vital because:

   - A) Participants' understanding and agreement may change over time.

   - B) It's a one-time requirement at the start of the trial.

   - C) It allows for the exclusion of non-compliant participants only.

   - D) Participants enjoy filling out paperwork.

7. Local ethics review is necessary to:

   - A) Create additional obstacles for trial sponsors.

   - B) Ensure trials meet both international and local ethical standards.

   - C) Standardize ethical considerations across all cultures.

   - D) Focus exclusively on international ethical standards.

8. Cultural competence training for trial teams helps in:

   - A) Minimizing the need for communication with participants.

   - B) Effectively interacting with participants from diverse backgrounds.

   - C) Ignoring cultural differences to streamline trial processes.

   - D) Promoting a one-size-fits-all approach to trial conduct.

9. Equitable access to trial participation aims to:

   - A) Limit participation to certain demographic groups.

   - B) Ensure all populations have an opportunity to participate.

   - C) Focus recruitment efforts on easily accessible participants.

   - D) Disregard the needs of underserved or marginalized populations.

10. Effective communication in global trials is characterized by:

- A) Reliance on technical and medical jargon.

- B) One-way communication from the trial team to participants.

- C) Clear, jargon-free language tailored to the audience.

- D) Avoiding the translation of trial documents.

Answers:

1. B) Ensuring respect for local norms and participant engagement.

2. C) Respect for persons, beneficence, and justice.

3. C) Adjusting to cultural norms and ensuring comprehension.

4. B) Building trust and fostering collaboration with local communities.

5. B) Providing equitable access and benefit sharing with participant communities.

6. A) Participants' understanding and agreement may change over time.

7. B) Ensure trials meet both international and local ethical standards.

8. B) Effectively interacting with participants from diverse backgrounds.

9. B) Ensure all populations have an opportunity to participate.

10. C) Clear, jargon-free language tailored to the audience.

Chapter 14: Innovations in Clinical Trial Design

14.1 Adaptive Trial Designs

Adaptive trial designs represent a significant innovation in clinical research, offering flexibility to modify trial parameters based on interim data analysis without compromising the study's integrity or validity. This approach can lead to more efficient and potentially faster trials, optimizing resources and potentially improving outcomes for participants. Here's an overview of adaptive trial designs:

Definition and Key Features:

- **Adaptive Design:** A trial design that allows for specified modifications to the trial and/or statistical procedures after its initiation without undermining its validity and integrity. Key modifications can include dosage adjustments, sample size recalculations, and eligibility criteria changes.

- **Pre-specified Adaptations:** Any adaptations are pre-specified in the trial protocol, detailing the conditions under which changes can be made, the decision-making process, and the statistical methods to be used for interim analyses.

Benefits of Adaptive Trial Designs:

1. **Increased Efficiency:** Allows for the early termination of ineffective treatment arms, focusing resources on more promising interventions.

2. **Enhanced Flexibility:** Provides the ability to adjust trial parameters in response to interim data, potentially leading to more effective and safer treatments being identified sooner.

3. **Improved Participant Safety:** Facilitates quicker adjustments based on safety data, minimizing participant exposure to ineffective or harmful treatments.

4. **Better Resource Utilization:** Potentially reduces the number of participants needed and the overall duration of the trial by adapting based on interim findings.

5. **Data-Driven Decisions:** Supports making informed decisions during the trial, enhancing the probability of success by adapting to emerging data.

Types of Adaptations in Clinical Trials:

- **Sample Size Re-Estimation:** Adjusting the sample size based on interim analysis to ensure the trial is adequately powered to detect treatment effects.

- **Dose Adjustment:** Modifying dosage levels in response to safety and efficacy data to identify optimal treatment regimens.

- **Seamless Phase Transition:** Combining phases of clinical development (e.g., Phase I/II or Phase II/III) to streamline the trial process.

- **Drop-the-Loser Designs:** Discontinuing less effective treatment arms based on interim results, focusing on more promising therapies.

- **Biomarker-Adaptive Design:** Utilizing biomarker data to select participants more likely to benefit from the treatment, improving the precision of the trial outcomes.

Challenges and Considerations:

- **Statistical Complexity:** Requires sophisticated statistical methods and careful planning to ensure the validity of the trial results.

- **Regulatory Acceptance:** Must be accepted by regulatory authorities, necessitating clear communication and justification of the adaptive design chosen.

- **Operational Demands:** Poses challenges in trial management and execution, requiring robust data management systems and real-time data analysis capabilities.

- **Transparency and Ethics:** Maintaining transparency about the adaptive process and ensuring ethical considerations are addressed throughout the trial.

Adaptive trial designs represent a paradigm shift in clinical research, offering a pathway to more dynamic, responsive, and patient-centered trials. However, their successful implementation demands thorough planning, clear protocols, and close collaboration among clinical researchers, statisticians, and regulatory authorities.

14.2 Patient-Centric Approaches

Patient-centric approaches in clinical trial design prioritize the needs, preferences, and overall experience of participants. By focusing on the patient's perspective, these approaches aim to enhance participation and retention rates, improve data quality, and ensure the relevance of research outcomes to patient needs. Here's how patient-centricity is being integrated into clinical trials:

1. Involving Patients in Trial Design:

- **Patient Advisory Panels:** Engage patients or patient advocacy groups early in the trial design process to gain insights into their needs and preferences. This involvement can inform various aspects of the trial, including protocol development, informed consent processes, and outcome measures that are meaningful to patients.

- **Feedback Loops:** Establish mechanisms for ongoing patient feedback throughout the trial to make adjustments that improve the patient experience.

2. Simplifying Trial Participation:

- **Decentralized Trials:** Utilize telemedicine, mobile health technologies, and local healthcare providers to allow patients to participate in trials from their homes or local communities, reducing the need for travel to trial sites.

- **Flexible Scheduling:** Offer flexible visit schedules and remote monitoring options to accommodate participants' daily routines and commitments.

3. Enhancing Informed Consent:

- **Clear Communication:** Use plain language and visual aids to ensure informed consent documents are easily understandable for participants, helping them make informed decisions about their participation.

- **Continuous Consent:** Treat informed consent as an ongoing process, providing participants with updates about the trial and re-confirming their consent as necessary, especially when there are significant changes to the trial protocol.

4. Improving Participant Support and Engagement:

- **Dedicated Support:** Provide participants with access to dedicated support teams or liaisons who can answer questions, address concerns, and offer assistance throughout the trial.

- **Engagement Activities:** Implement engagement strategies, such as regular updates on trial progress, educational materials about the condition being studied, and community-building activities, to keep participants informed and involved.

5. Addressing Diversity and Inclusivity:

- **Broad Inclusion Criteria:** Design trials with inclusion criteria that reflect the diversity of the patient population affected by the condition being studied, ensuring the trial findings are applicable to a wide patient base.

- **Cultural Competence:** Train trial staff in cultural competence to effectively communicate and interact with participants from diverse backgrounds, ensuring that all participants feel respected and valued.

6. Focusing on Patient-Reported Outcomes:

- **Relevant Outcomes:** Incorporate patient-reported outcomes (PROs) as primary or secondary endpoints to capture the impact of interventions on patients' quality of life, symptoms, and overall well-being from their perspective.

- **Technology Integration:** Use electronic PRO (ePRO) tools and apps to facilitate real-time, convenient reporting of outcomes by patients.

Patient-centric approaches are transforming clinical trial design by ensuring that trials are more accessible, relevant, and engaging for participants. This focus on the patient perspective not only enhances the ethical conduct of research but also contributes to the generation of meaningful and applicable scientific evidence.

14.3 The Future of Clinical Trial Methodologies

The landscape of clinical trial methodologies is rapidly evolving, driven by technological advancements, the increasing importance of patient-centric approaches, and the need for more efficient and flexible research frameworks. This evolution aims to address the complexities of modern healthcare challenges, accelerate the development of innovative treatments, and ensure that research outcomes are both scientifically robust and highly relevant to patient needs. Here's a glimpse into the future of clinical trial methodologies:

1. Integration of Real-World Data (RWD) and Real-World Evidence (RWE):

- **Expanding Evidence Base:** The use of RWD (healthcare data from electronic health records, insurance claims, patient registries, and wearable devices) and RWE (evidence derived from analyzing RWD) is set to expand, informing trial designs, patient recruitment strategies, and regulatory decisions. This integration can make trials more reflective of real-world patient populations and treatment effects.

2. Artificial Intelligence and Machine Learning:

- **Data Analysis and Prediction:** AI and machine learning algorithms will increasingly be used to analyze complex datasets, identify patterns, predict trial outcomes, and optimize study designs. This can lead to more targeted and efficient trials, especially in identifying biomarkers for disease and predicting patient responses to treatments.

3. Decentralized and Virtual Trials:

- **Increasing Accessibility:** The move towards decentralized and virtual trials, which reduce or eliminate the need for in-person visits, is expected to continue. This shift not only increases trial accessibility for diverse patient populations but also enhances flexibility in data collection and participant monitoring.

4. Patient Engagement Platforms:

- **Enhanced Communication:** Digital platforms and mobile apps that facilitate direct communication between researchers and participants will become more prevalent. These tools can support informed consent processes, real-time data collection (ePROs), and provide participants with information and support, enhancing engagement and adherence.

5. Adaptive and Platform Trial Designs:

- **Flexibility and Efficiency:** The future will see broader adoption of adaptive trial designs, allowing for modifications based on interim data analysis, and platform trials, which test multiple treatments within the same overarching framework. These designs offer flexibility, efficiency, and the ability to rapidly integrate new treatments or hypotheses.

6. Focus on Diversity and Inclusivity:

- **Reflecting Real-World Populations:** There will be a greater emphasis on ensuring clinical trial populations reflect the diversity of patients affected by the condition under study. This includes efforts to overcome barriers to participation for underrepresented groups, ensuring that trial results are generalizable and applicable to all segments of the population.

7. Enhanced Collaboration and Data Sharing:

- **Global Partnerships:** The future of clinical trials will likely involve more collaborative models between academic institutions, industry, healthcare providers, and patient organizations. Enhanced data sharing and transparency among stakeholders can accelerate the generation of knowledge and the approval of new treatments.

8. Regulatory Evolution:

- **Keeping Pace with Innovation:** Regulatory frameworks and guidelines will continue to evolve to keep pace with technological advancements and methodological innovations in clinical trial design. This includes the development of new guidelines for the use of digital health technologies, RWE, and patient-centric outcome measures.

The future of clinical trial methodologies is marked by innovation, flexibility, and an unwavering focus on delivering meaningful health outcomes for patients. As these new approaches are implemented, the clinical research ecosystem will become more efficient, inclusive, and capable of addressing the pressing health challenges of the 21st century.

14.4 Exercise: 10 MCQs with Answers at the End

Multiple Choice Questions:

1. What is a key benefit of integrating Real-World Data (RWD) into clinical trial designs?

  - A) Decreasing the trial's relevance to everyday practice.

  - B) Making trials less reflective of the general population.

  - C) Enhancing the evidence base and informing patient recruitment.

  - D) Complicating data analysis processes.

2. How can artificial intelligence (AI) and machine learning revolutionize clinical trials?

   - A) By reducing the need for data.

   - B) Through optimizing study designs and predicting outcomes.

   - C) Eliminating the role of human researchers.

   - D) Decreasing the accuracy of data analysis.

3. What characterizes decentralized and virtual trials?

   - A) Requirement for more in-person visits.

   - B) Reduced trial accessibility for participants.

   - C) Increased trial accessibility and flexibility.

   - D) Longer durations for data collection.

4. Patient engagement platforms in clinical trials are designed to:

   - A) Limit patient communication with researchers.

   - B) Enhance communication and support informed consent processes.

   - C) Discourage real-time data collection.

   - D) Increase the complexity of trial participation for patients.

5. Adaptive trial designs allow for:

  - A) No modifications based on interim data.

  - B) Decreased trial efficiency and flexibility.

   - C) Specified modifications to the trial based on interim data analysis.

  - D) Unplanned changes at any point during the trial.

6. The future of clinical trials aims to improve diversity and inclusivity by:

  - A) Only focusing on majority populations.

  - B) Reflecting the diversity of patients affected by the condition under study.

   - C) Ignoring barriers to participation for underrepresented groups.

  - D) Limiting the geographical locations of trials.

7. Enhanced collaboration and data sharing in future clinical trials will likely involve:

  - A) Decreased transparency among stakeholders.

  - B) More siloed research efforts.

  - C) Collaborative models and global partnerships.

  - D) Reducing the pace of innovation in trial methodologies.

8. What will be necessary as clinical trial methodologies evolve and incorporate new technologies?

   - A) Simplified regulatory guidelines.

   - B) Less focus on patient-centric outcomes.

- C) Regulatory frameworks evolving to keep pace with innovation.

   - D) Discouragement of digital health technology use.

9. The use of ePRO tools in future clinical trials facilitates:

   - A) Less accurate patient-reported outcome collection.

   - B) Real-time, convenient reporting of outcomes by patients.

   - C) Decreased patient engagement in the trial.

   - D) Increased burden on trial participants.

10. Platform trial designs are significant because they:

   - A) Limit the ability to test multiple treatments simultaneously.

   - B) Increase the complexity and cost with no added benefit.

   - C) Offer flexibility and the ability to integrate new treatments rapidly.

   - D) Focus exclusively on a single hypothesis without adaptation.

Answers:

1. C) Enhancing the evidence base and informing patient recruitment.

2. B) Through optimizing study designs and predicting outcomes.

3. C) Increased trial accessibility and flexibility.

4. B) Enhance communication and support informed consent processes.

5. C) Specified modifications to the trial based on interim data analysis.

6. B) Reflecting the diversity of patients affected by the condition under study.

7. C) Collaborative models and global partnerships.

8. C) Regulatory frameworks evolving to keep pace with innovation.

9. B) Real-time, convenient reporting of outcomes by patients.

10. C) Offer flexibility and the ability to integrate new treatments rapidly.

Chapter 15: Career Development for Clinical Trial Managers

15.1 Navigating Career Paths in Clinical Research

A career in clinical research offers a range of pathways and opportunities for professional growth and development. Clinical trial managers play a crucial role in the research ecosystem, overseeing the execution of trials, ensuring compliance with regulatory standards, and contributing to the advancement of medical knowledge. Here's a guide to navigating career paths in clinical research:

1. Understanding the Clinical Research Landscape:

- **Diverse Roles:** The field encompasses a variety of roles, including clinical research coordinators (CRCs), clinical research associates (CRAs), data managers, regulatory affairs specialists, and project managers, each contributing differently to trial success.

- **Employment Settings:** Opportunities exist across pharmaceutical companies, biotech firms, contract research organizations (CROs), academic research institutions, and healthcare providers.

2. Building a Foundation:

- **Education:** A bachelor's degree in life sciences, nursing, pharmacy, public health, or a related field is typically the minimum requirement. Advanced degrees (Master's, PhD) or specialized certifications (e.g., Certified Clinical Research Professional, CCRP) can enhance prospects.

- **Entry-Level Experience:** Gaining experience as a CRC or a research assistant can provide valuable insights into trial operations and patient interactions, forming a strong foundation for a career in trial management.

3. Developing Skills and Expertise:

- **Core Competencies:** Essential skills include project management, regulatory compliance, data analysis, and ethical considerations. Soft skills such as communication, leadership, and problem-solving are equally important.

- **Continuing Education:** Stay abreast of industry trends, regulatory changes, and innovations in trial design by pursuing continuous education opportunities, attending workshops, and participating in professional organizations.

4. Advancement Opportunities:

- **Career Ladder:** Career progression can lead from coordinating or assisting roles to trial management, project leadership, and eventually to senior positions such as director of clinical operations or vice president of clinical research.

- **Specialization:** Consider specializing in certain therapeutic areas, regulatory affairs, data management, or patient recruitment strategies to distinguish your expertise and value.

5. Networking and Professional Development:

- **Industry Associations:** Join professional associations such as the Association of Clinical Research Professionals (ACRP) or the Society for Clinical Trials (SCT) to access resources, training, and networking opportunities.

- **Mentorship:** Seek mentorship from experienced professionals in the field. Mentors can provide guidance, career advice, and introductions to opportunities.

6. Considerations for Career Growth:

- **Flexibility:** Be open to relocating or changing employment settings to gain diverse experiences and advance your career.

- **Leadership Roles:** Aspire to leadership positions by developing strategic thinking, people management skills, and a thorough understanding of the clinical research landscape.

7. Keeping an Eye on the Future:

- **Emerging Trends:** Stay informed about emerging trends such as decentralized trials, digital health technologies, and patient-centric approaches to position yourself as a forward-thinking professional in the field.

Navigating a career in clinical research requires a blend of education, experience, and continuous learning. By building a broad skill set, specializing in areas of interest, and engaging with the professional community, clinical trial managers can achieve rewarding careers that contribute significantly to advancing healthcare and patient outcomes.

15.2 Skills and Competencies for Advancement

Advancing in the field of clinical trial management requires a combination of technical knowledge, soft skills, and a proactive approach to career development. Here are essential skills and competencies that clinical trial managers should cultivate for career advancement:

1. Technical Expertise:

- **Regulatory Knowledge:** Deep understanding of regulatory requirements and ethical guidelines in clinical research, including FDA regulations, ICH-GCP, and EMA guidelines.

- **Clinical Trial Operations:** Proficiency in all phases of trial operations, from study design and protocol development to data management and reporting.

- **Data Analysis and Interpretation:** Ability to analyze and interpret clinical data, including statistical analysis skills and familiarity with data management systems.

2. Project Management Skills:

- **Planning and Organization:** Strong project planning and organizational skills to manage multiple aspects of clinical trials efficiently.

- **Risk Management:** Ability to identify potential risks in trial execution and develop strategies to mitigate these risks.

- **Budget Management:** Competence in managing trial budgets, understanding financial aspects, and ensuring cost-effective trial execution.

3. Leadership and Team Management:

- **Communication:** Excellent communication skills for effective interaction with trial teams, stakeholders, and participants. This includes the ability to convey complex information clearly and concisely.

- **Team Leadership:** Strong leadership skills to motivate, guide, and manage diverse trial teams, including conflict resolution and team-building abilities.

- **Decision-Making:** Sound decision-making skills, with the ability to make informed choices under pressure and adapt to changing circumstances.

4. Patient-Centric Approach:

- **Ethical Considerations:** A deep commitment to ethical standards and patient safety, ensuring that trials are conducted with the utmost respect for participants.

- **Patient Engagement:** Skills in patient engagement and recruitment, understanding patient needs and preferences, and incorporating patient-centric approaches in trial design.

5. Adaptability and Continuous Learning:

- **Adaptability:** Flexibility to adapt to new technologies, methodologies, and regulatory changes in the fast-evolving field of clinical research.

- **Continuous Learning:** Commitment to lifelong learning through professional development courses, certifications, and staying updated with industry trends and innovations.

6. Technology Proficiency:

- **Digital Tools and Platforms:** Proficiency in using clinical trial management systems (CTMS), electronic data capture (EDC) systems, and other digital tools to enhance trial efficiency.

- **Emerging Technologies:** Openness to adopting emerging technologies, such as decentralized trial platforms, wearable devices, and artificial intelligence applications in clinical research.

7. Networking and Professional Development:

- **Professional Networking:** Active engagement in professional organizations, conferences, and workshops to build a network of contacts, share knowledge, and identify career opportunities.

- **Mentorship:** Both seeking mentorship from experienced professionals and mentoring junior colleagues to contribute to the professional growth within the clinical research community.

Developing these skills and competencies can significantly enhance a clinical trial manager's ability to lead successful trials, contribute to medical advancements, and progress to higher leadership roles within the field of clinical research.

15.3 Continuing Education and Professional Development

In the rapidly evolving field of clinical research, ongoing education and professional development are pivotal for individuals aiming to advance their careers and enhance their effectiveness as clinical trial managers. This commitment to learning ensures professionals stay abreast of the latest methodologies, regulatory changes, and technological advancements. Here's how to approach continuing education and professional development in this dynamic field:

1. Formal Educational Programs:

- **Advanced Degrees:** Pursuing an advanced degree in a relevant field such as public health, epidemiology, or bioinformatics can deepen your expertise and open up opportunities for higher-level positions.

- **Specialized Courses:** Enroll in courses that focus on specific aspects of clinical trials, such as regulatory affairs, data management, or biostatistics, to build specialized knowledge that can differentiate you in the job market.

2. Certification Programs:

- Engage in certification programs designed for clinical research professionals. These programs often cover core areas like trial management, ethical conduct of research, and regulatory compliance, providing a recognized credential that can enhance your professional credibility.

3. Workshops, Seminars, and Conferences:

- Participate in industry workshops, seminars, and conferences to gain insights into current trends, best practices, and future directions in clinical research. These events also offer valuable networking opportunities with peers and leaders in the field.

4. Online Learning Platforms:

- Leverage online learning platforms that offer courses and webinars on a wide range of topics relevant to clinical research. Many of these platforms provide flexible learning options that can fit into a busy professional schedule.

5. Professional Associations:

- Join professional associations related to clinical research. Membership often includes access to exclusive resources, educational materials, and events that can support your professional development. Additionally, these associations can provide opportunities to contribute to the field, such as through committee involvement or publication in professional journals.

6. Peer Learning and Networking:

- Engage in peer learning opportunities by participating in discussion forums, study groups, or mentorship programs. Sharing experiences and challenges with colleagues can provide practical insights and enhance your problem-solving skills.

- Build and maintain a professional network that includes a diverse range of roles within clinical research. Networking can open doors to new opportunities and collaborations.

7. Self-directed Learning:

- Stay informed about the latest research, regulatory updates, and innovations in clinical trial design by reading professional journals, attending webinars, and following thought leaders in the field.

- Reflect on your own experiences and identify areas for improvement. Setting personal learning objectives and seeking out resources to meet these goals can drive your professional growth.

8. Ethical and Cultural Competence:

- Ensure that your professional development includes a focus on ethical considerations in clinical research and cultural competence. Understanding the ethical frameworks that guide clinical research and being sensitive to cultural differences are essential for conducting global and diverse trials.

Continuous education and professional development are essential strategies for clinical trial managers seeking to excel in their careers. By embracing a multifaceted approach to learning and staying engaged with the broader clinical research community, professionals can ensure they remain effective, relevant, and capable of contributing to advancements in healthcare research.

15.4 Exercise: 10 MCQs with Answers at the End

Multiple Choice Questions:

1. What is a fundamental reason for clinical trial managers to pursue continuing education?

   - A) To fulfill time management requirements.

   - B) To stay abreast of advancements and regulatory changes in clinical research.

   - C) To minimize interaction with colleagues.

   - D) For the sole purpose of salary increment.

2. Advanced degrees in clinical research can:

   - A) Limit career opportunities in clinical trials.

   - B) Provide deeper expertise and open up higher-level position opportunities.

   - C) Decrease a professional's marketability.

   - D) Discourage lifelong learning.

3. Certification programs for clinical research professionals are designed to:

   - A) Decrease the individual's credibility in the field.

- B) Enhance professional credibility through recognized credentials.

   - C) Overwhelm professionals with unnecessary information.

   - D) Isolate professionals from practical experiences.

4. Attending industry conferences and workshops can primarily help professionals:

   - A) Avoid networking opportunities.

   - B) Gain insights into current trends and best practices in clinical research.

   - C) Limit exposure to new methodologies.

   - D) Focus solely on past achievements in the field.

5. Online learning platforms offer courses in clinical research to:

- A) Discourage flexibility and self-paced learning.

- B) Provide flexible learning options for busy professionals.

- C) Undermine traditional educational methods.

- D) Decrease accessibility to specialized knowledge.

6. Membership in professional associations related to clinical research can provide:

- A) Limited access to educational materials and events.

- B) Decreased opportunities for professional networking.

- C) Access to exclusive resources and educational materials.

- D) An environment that discourages professional contribution.

7. Peer learning opportunities in clinical research can:

- A) Prevent professionals from sharing experiences and challenges.

- B) Provide practical insights and enhance problem-solving skills.

- C) Encourage professionals to work in isolation.

- D) Discourage the development of a professional network.

8. Self-directed learning is important for clinical trial managers because it:

   - A) Encourages complacency in professional roles.

   - B) Allows professionals to identify and pursue their own learning objectives.

   - C) Decreases awareness of industry advancements.

   - D) Limits exposure to diverse perspectives in clinical research.

9. Focusing on ethical considerations and cultural competence is essential because:

   - A) It limits the manager's ability to conduct global trials.

   - B) It is irrelevant to modern clinical research practices.

   - C) It ensures research is conducted responsibly and is sensitive to cultural differences.

   - D) Ethical considerations have little impact on trial outcomes.

10. Continuous education and professional development in clinical research:

   - A) Are unnecessary for experienced professionals.

   - B) Can drive professional growth and contribute to advancements in healthcare research.

   - C) Discourage innovation in trial design and methodologies.

   - D) Are solely focused on theoretical knowledge.

Answers:

1. B) To stay abreast of advancements and regulatory changes in clinical research.

2. B) Provide deeper expertise and open up higher-level position opportunities.

3. B) Enhance professional credibility through recognized credentials.

4. B) Gain insights into current trends and best practices in clinical research.

5. B) Provide flexible learning options for busy professionals.

6. C) Access to exclusive resources and educational materials.

7. B) Provide practical insights and enhance problem-solving skills.

8. B) Allows professionals to identify and pursue their own learning objectives.

9. C) It ensures research is conducted responsibly and is sensitive to cultural differences.

10. B) Can drive professional growth and contribute to advancements in healthcare research.

Conclusion

As we conclude this comprehensive exploration of clinical trials, from their foundational principles and ethical considerations to the nuances of global trial conduct and the evolving landscape of trial methodologies, it's clear that the field of clinical research is both complex and dynamic. Key takeaways include the importance of ethical integrity, the value of stakeholder engagement, and the need for continuous professional development in navigating the challenges and opportunities inherent in clinical trial management.

The journey through various aspects of clinical trials underscores the critical role of innovation, patient-centricity, and effective communication in advancing medical knowledge and improving patient care. As the field continues to evolve with technological advancements and shifts towards more inclusive, flexible, and efficient trial designs, professionals within the clinical research ecosystem must remain agile, informed, and committed to ethical excellence.

For those embarking on or advancing within a career in clinical trial management, the landscape is rich with opportunities for impactful work that contributes to the betterment of global health outcomes. Embracing lifelong learning, fostering collaborations, and maintaining a steadfast focus on the welfare of trial participants are key to success and fulfillment in this vital field.

In closing, the realm of clinical trials is a testament to the collaborative efforts of countless individuals dedicated to the pursuit of scientific discovery and the betterment of human health. As we look to the future, let us carry forward the lessons learned, the innovations developed, and the ethical standards upheld, with a shared commitment to improving the lives of patients around the world.

*The best way to thank an author is
to
write a review.*